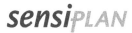

Malteser Arbeitsgruppe NFP

Natural & Safe: The Workbook
Family Planning with Sensiplan

Malteser
...weil Nähe zählt.

Natural & Safe: The Workbook
Family Planning with Sensiplan

ISBN 978-1-7336878-2-9 (soft cover)
ISBN 978-1-7336878-3-6 (e-book)

CycleForth publishes the English language editions of *Natural & Safe: The Handbook, Family Planning with Sensiplan* and *Natural & Safe: The Workbook, Family Planning with Sensiplan,* and coordinates provision of education in the Sensiplan method with Reply Ob/Gyn & Fertility. Please visit www.replyobgyn.com/services/sensiplan.

Malteser Arbeitsgruppe NFP is an interdisciplinary team that operates as part of Malteser Health Promotion and Prevention. Arbeitsgruppe NFP is focused on development of natural family planning ("NFP") and quality assurance in NFP consulting and training.

Original German title:
Arbeitsgruppe Natürliche Familienplanung (NFP), Natürlich und Sicher: Das Arbeitsheft,
10th revised edition 2015
© 2004, 2015 TRIAS Verlag in MVS Medizinverlage Stuttgart GmbH & Co. KG, Oswald-Hesse-Straße 50, 70469 Stuttgart, Germany
© 1st-6th edition, Ehrenwirth in der Verlagsgruppe lübbe GmbH & Co. KG

DISCLAIMER: Information in this book is for educational purposes only without representations or warranties of any kind, express or implied. Instruction with a certified fertility educator is recommended for those seeking to use Sensiplan for family planning. None of this information constitutes, or is a substitute for, professional medical advice, diagnosis, or treatment. A physician should be consulted for medical advice.

Malteser Arbeitsgruppe NFP

Natural & Safe: The Workbook
Family Planning with Sensiplan

-- Safe and effective family planning with Sensiplan™
-- With sample cycles from puberty to menopause

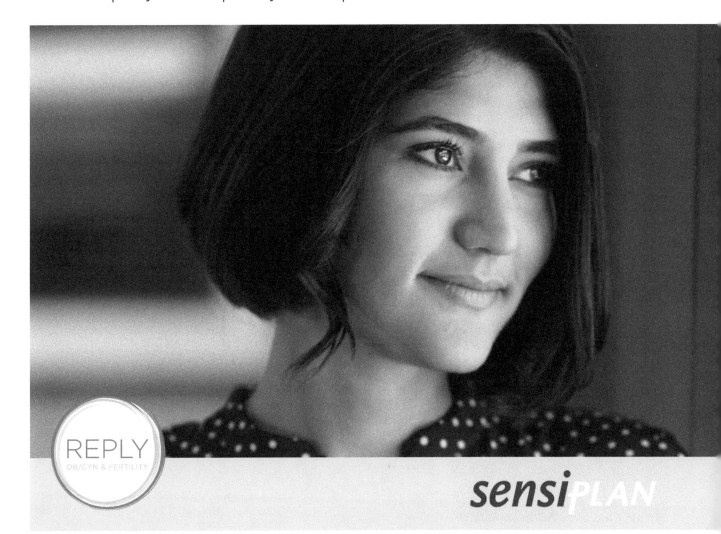

REPLY
OB/GYN & FERTILITY

*sensi*PLAN

Learning Sensiplan

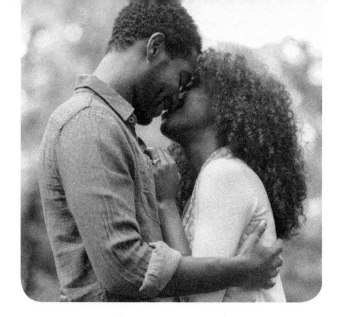

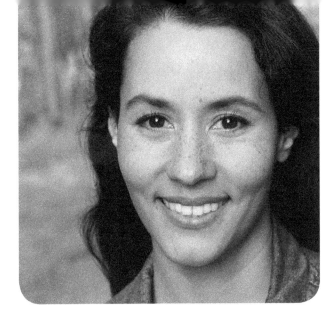

Foreword

Sensiplan is a fertility awareness-based method of family planning, known also as natural family planning ("NFP"). It was developed in Germany over a period of decades by the "Arbeitsgruppe NFP," or "NFP Working Group," at the international aid agency Malteser International, and with help from the German Ministry of Health.

Natural & Safe: The Handbook and *Natural & Safe: The Workbook* are two important Sensiplan resources, translated now for the first time in English. *The Handbook* describes the method and how it complements the function of a woman's body, while *The Workbook* provides practice charts, case examples, and specific instruction for using the method throughout various phases of life.

CycleForth LLC is the Des Moines, Iowa-based company that introduced Sensiplan in the United States in 2016, and now is making available the *Natural & Safe* companion texts. CycleForth specializes in development of cooperative and restorative health care products and services, and coordinates provision of Sensiplan and other fertility awareness-based methods through fertility educators at Reply Ob/Gyn & Fertility. For their decades of commitment to development of Sensiplan, we thank Malteser Arbeitsgruppe NFP. For their trainings in Sensiplan and many contributions to this project, we especially thank our German colleagues Dr. Ursula Sottong and Petra Klann-Heinen. For their work on this English translation and introducing Sensiplan in the U.S., we thank fertility educators Lori Hartley, Donna Zubrod, Emily Kennedy and Dr. Rachel Urrutia, and for her tireless efforts on graphics and layout of this text, we thank Barri Burch.

To learn more about Sensiplan's established record of effectiveness, or to inquire about learning the method with a certified fertility educator either in clinic or via telehealth, please contact:

Reply Ob/Gyn & Fertility
Sensiplan Instruction, Suite 105
7535 Carpenter Fire Station Road | Cary, NC 27519
919-230-2100 | info@replyobgyn.com | www.replyobgyn.com/services/sensiplan

For information about Sensiplan instruction offered globally, please contact:

Malteser Arbeitsgruppe
SENSIPLAN
Erna-Schefflerstr.2 | 51103 Cologne
www.nfp-online.de | www.sensiplan.de

Preface

Sensiplan is a natural method of family planning developed and scientifically evaluated by the Malteser Arbeitsgruppe, or "Working Group," for Natural Family Planning. It has been established through prospective clinical research conducted over a period of many years and published in peer-reviewed medical journals.

Users can begin using Sensiplan during the first cycle, however, the user must understand the Senisplan rules and feel comfortable making and recording observations. A detailed overview of the Sensiplan method and rules are found in the companion book, *Natural & Safe: The Handbook, Family Planning with Sensiplan.*

This *Workbook* includes a wide range of life situations and cycle examples a woman may experience over the course of her lifetime, and is an important prerequisite for the effective and safe application of Sensiplan.

Natural & Safe: The Workbook was first published in German in 1988, and was completely revised for the first time ten years later. This current edition, now translated into English for the first time, relies on more than 20 years of teaching experience with Arbeitsgruppe Sensiplan and the observation of 42,000 cycles from which data were collected and scientifically evaluated.

We would like to extend our thanks to Dr. Siegfried Baur and Dr. Ursula Sottong, who, alongside Regina Jäger, have revised the *Workbook* and given it a new layout. We also would like to give our special thanks to everyone who has enabled the work of the Arbeitsgruppe Sensiplan task force, and who has supported the group in various ways, as well as the men and women who have provided us with their experiences and cycle charts.

Malteser Arbeitsgruppe NFP
Sensiplan
Cologne, April 2012

Introduction

Sensiplan is an established method of fertility awareness, or natural family planning ("NFP"), by which women monitor physical signs that change throughout their reproductive cycles. Understanding these signs allows a woman to identify her fertile and infertile days and include:

• Changes in Body Temperature

• Changes in Cervical Mucus

• The Position of the Cervix

A woman who can interpret these signs knows when in her cycle pregnancy is possible, and when it is not. She can plan intercourse with her partner depending on whether or not she is trying to conceive. The use of Sensiplan requires cooperation between both partners.

How does Sensiplan work?

For pregnancy to occur, the egg and sperm must meet. The egg is only released once per cycle, and can survive up to 24 hours. Sperm, on the other hand, can survive in the female body for several days around the time of ovulation. During this time the first-morning temperature (basal body temperature), cervical mucus, and the cervix undergo observable changes. Women using Sensiplan learn to monitor these physical signs every day, record them on a "cycle chart," and then evaluate them based on easy-to-apply rules. Sensiplan allows a woman to identify her fertile time and to actively choose whether or not to try to achieve or avoid pregnancy in any given cycle.

Basal Body Temperature

If you track your basal body temperature throughout a cycle, you will see that there are two temperature phases. Before ovulation, body temperature is slightly lower. Around ovulation, a woman's basal body temperature noticeably rises. This rise in temperature allows a woman to identify clearly the beginning of the infertile time after ovulation.

Cervical Mucus

Glands in the cervix excrete cervical mucus of varying quality and quantity during a cycle. Generally, women do not notice cervical mucus until a few days after menstrual bleeding stops.

Mucus is initially thick, partially sticky and creamy, and often has a whitish color. The closer the woman is to ovulation, the more cervical mucus is produced, and the more liquid and transparent it becomes - almost like raw egg white. This consistency allows sperm to pass through the cervix and survive for several days in the womb. After ovulation, the cervical mucus thickens again, seals the neck of the womb with a mucus plug, and is again impenetrable to sperm.

The Cervix

There is another physical sign by which a woman can observe whether or not she is in a fertile time: changes in the position and feeling of the cervix. By regularly feeling the cervix, a woman can tell how the position, firmness, and opening of the cervix changes during the cycle. After menstruation, the cervix is closed and hard, and it drops into the vagina. As she gets closer to ovulation, the cervix softens, opens, and slightly rises. After ovulation, the cervix closes again, becomes hard, and drops lower into the vagina.

Sensiplan –
The symptothermal method

This method derives its name from observing a combination of *symptoms* (cervical mucus or cervix) and basal body *temperature*: the symptothermal method. For Sensiplan to be reliable, temperature values and cervical mucus patterns must be evaluated and interpreted according to precise rules. These detailed rules allow the fertile time to be clearly identified. When used consistently Sensiplan can be, as current studies confirm, as reliable as contraceptive methods such as the birth control pill. Additionally, Sensiplan has no harmful side effects.

How can women and men learn Sensiplan?

There are two ways to learn: either by independent study using the books *Natural & Safe: The Handbook* and *Natural & Safe: The Workbook,* or by using the books along with the help of certified Sensiplan instructors. Experience has shown that having expert support during the initial learning phase leads to improved use of the rules and increases personal satisfaction with the method.

Although learning time varies among users, many women report increased confidence in using the method after completing three charted cycles. The method first teaches how to make self-observations, and then how to use the Sensiplan rules to identify the beginning and end of the fertile phase.

Also, special situations are discussed including how to recognize pregnancy using information collected from the chart. Experience has shown that almost all couples are able to independently and safely use Sensiplan after three cycles without further instruction.

About this workbook

This *Workbook* supplements the manual *Natural & Safe: The Handbook, Family Planning with Sensiplan* (CycleForth 2019). It contains examples and practice cycles, which can help users learn to use Sensiplan. The *Workbook* is divided into four sections. Each chapter builds on the information given in the previous chapter. In the first three chapters, there are plenty of exercises with solutions and detailed explanations of the Sensiplan rules. The fourth chapter contains sample cycles of special life circumstances, such as trying to conceive after discontinuing hormonal contraceptives.

Finally, rules are summarized at the end of this *Workbook* in the section titled **Sensiplan at-a-glance** on pages 165-167.

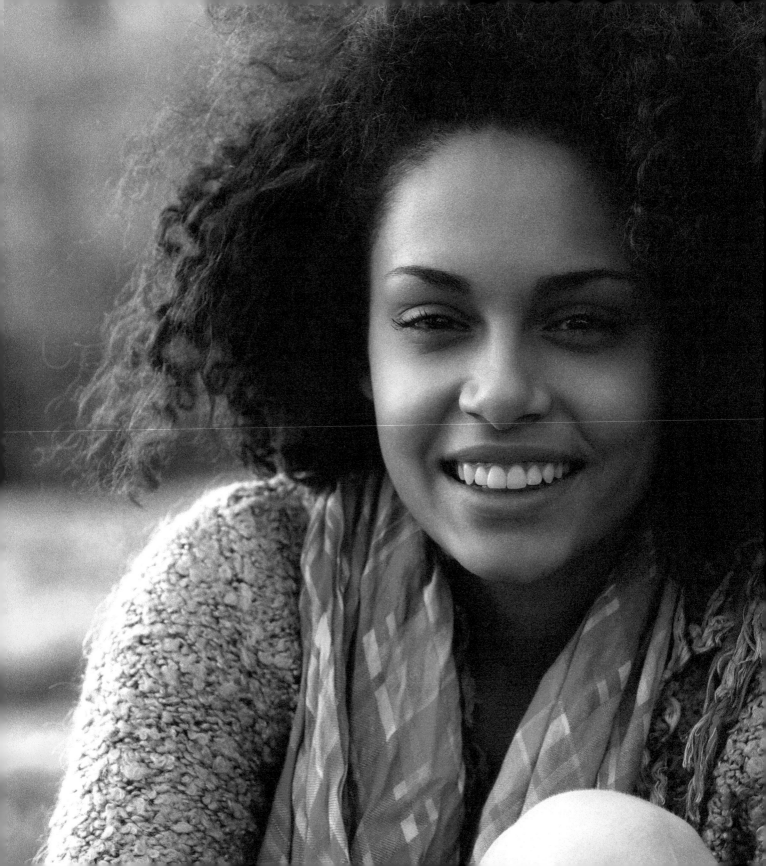

Chapter 1:

Observing signs of fertility

For the safe and reliable use of natural family planning, it is essential to observe and record physical changes during the female cycle. This section explains step by step how and when to make and record your observations.

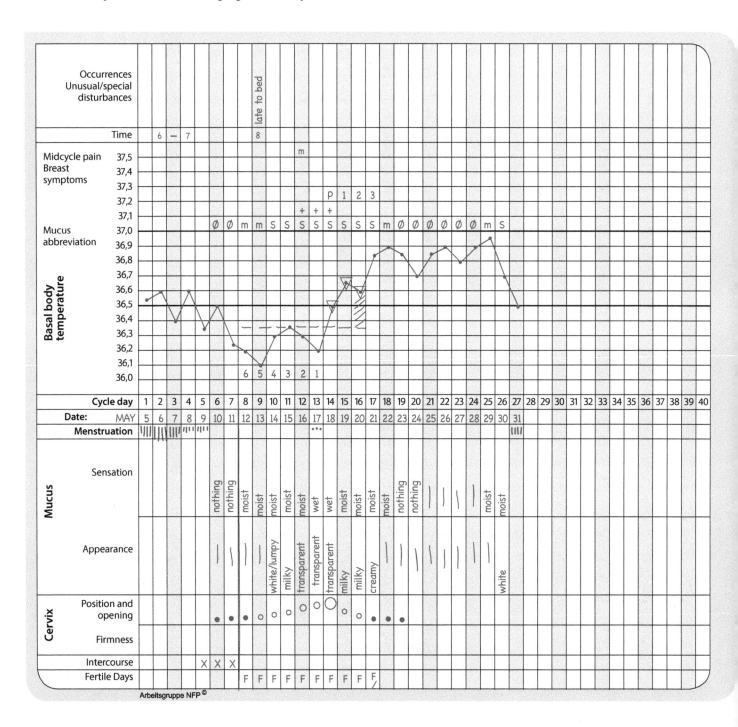

Arbeitsgruppe NFP ©

Observing and recording signs of fertility

While changes in basal body temperature and cervical mucus (or cervix position and feeling) are the primary signs used in Sensiplan, other signs can contribute to understanding a woman's fertility. These signs include mid-cycle pain and breast symptoms.

All observations are recorded on a cycle chart and evaluated. The cycle chart is like a personal diary and should include signs of fertility and other factors that could affect observing and interpreting the chart.

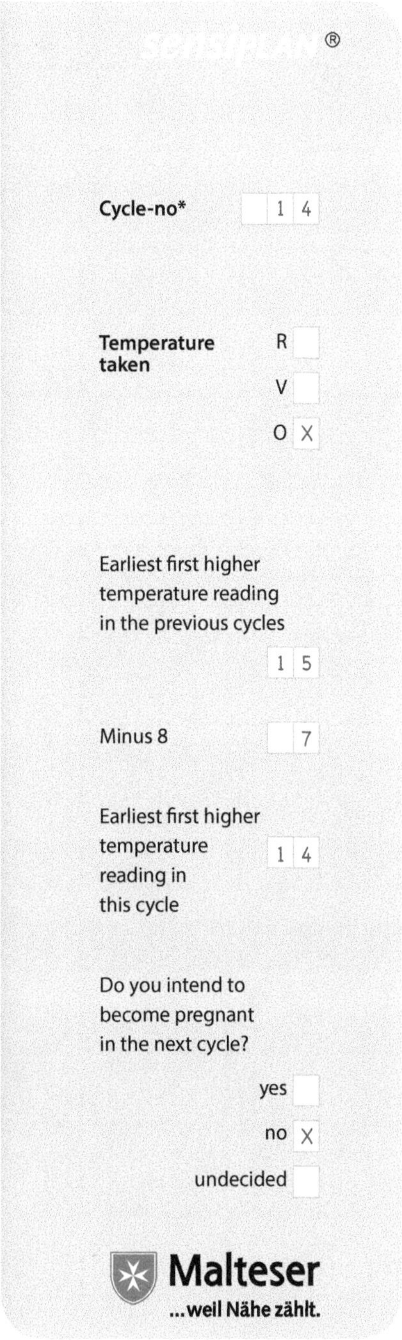
SENSIPLAN®

Cycle-no* 1 4

Temperature taken R ☐ V ☐ O X

Earliest first higher temperature reading in the previous cycles 1 5

Minus 8 7

Earliest first higher temperature reading in this cycle 1 4

Do you intend to become pregnant in the next cycle?
yes ☐
no X
undecided ☐

Malteser ...weil Nähe zählt.

Figure 1: Example of a completed cycle chart from an experienced user in the 14th cycle of using Sensiplan

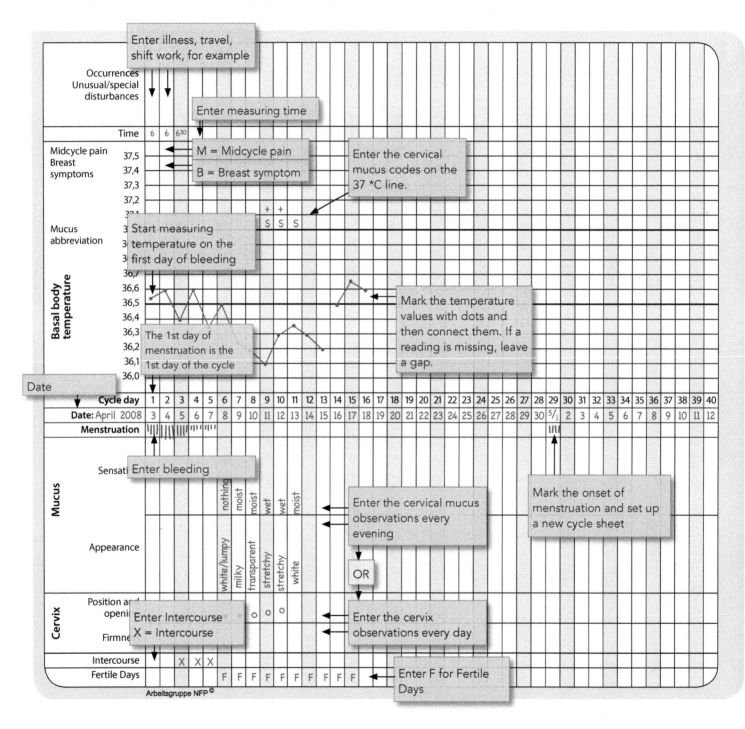

Enter illness, travel, shift work, for example

Occurrences
Unusual/special
disturbances

Enter measuring time

Time — 6 6 6³⁰

Midcycle pain
Breast
symptoms
37,5 — M = Midcycle pain
37,4 — B = Breast symptom
37,3
37,2

Enter the cervical mucus codes on the 37 *C line.

Mucus
abbreviation — Start measuring temperature on the first day of bleeding

36,7
Basal body temperature
36,6
36,5
36,4
36,3 — The 1st day of menstruation is the 1st day of the cycle
36,2
36,1
36,0

Mark the temperature values with dots and then connect them. If a reading is missing, leave a gap.

Date

Cycle day	1	2	3	4	5	6	7	8	9	10	11	12	13	14	15	16	17	18	19	20	21	22	23	24	25	26	27	28	29	30	31	32	33	34	35	36	37	38	39	40
Date: April 2008	3	4	5	6	7	8	9	10	11	12	13	14	15	16	17	18	19	20	21	22	23	24	25	26	27	28	29	30	⁵/₁	2	3	4	5	6	7	8	9	10	11	12

Menstruation

Mark the onset of menstruation and set up a new cycle sheet

Mucus

Sensation — Enter bleeding

nothing / moist / moist / wet / wet / moist

Appearance

white/lumpy / milky / transparent / stretchy / stretchy / white

Enter the cervical mucus observations every evening

OR

Cervix

Position and opening — Enter Intercourse X = Intercourse

Firmness

Enter the cervix observations every day

Intercourse — X X X

Fertile Days — F F F F F F F F F F

Enter F for Fertile Days

Arbeitsgruppe NFP ©

The cycle chart

The cycle chart looks more complicated than it is. See Fig. 2 for a sample cycle chart with an explanation of entries.

The cycle chart begins with the first day of menstruation, which is noted on the row marked "Date."

Bleeding is entered on the row marked "Menstruation" by using longer or shorter lines, or dots to indicate how heavy bleeding is.

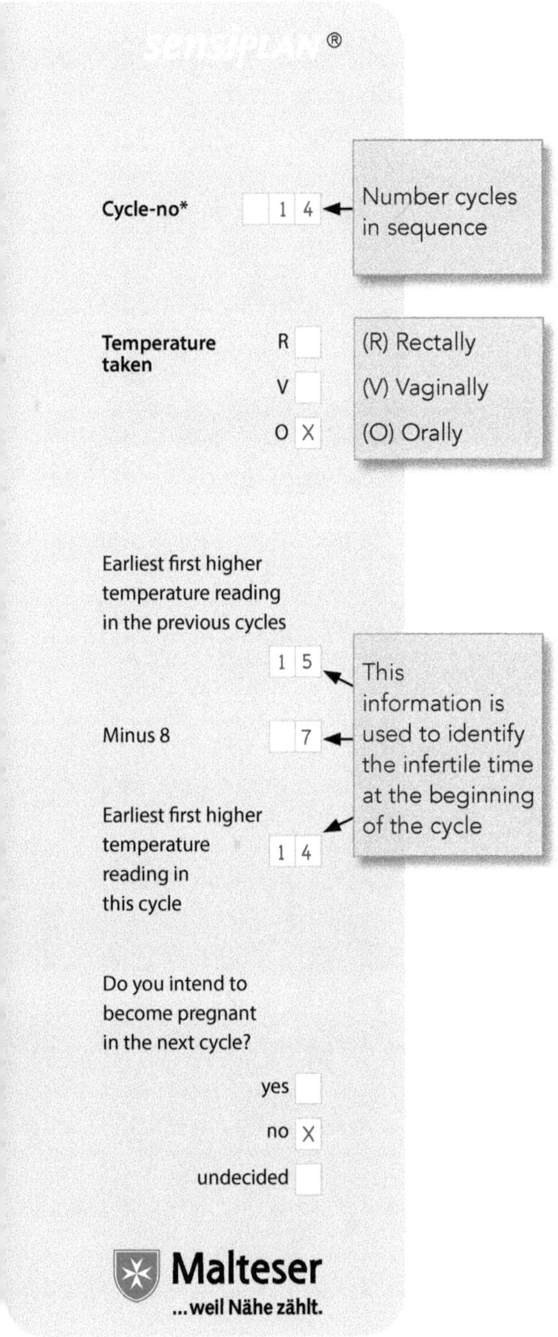

SENSIPLAN ®

| Cycle-no* | 1 | 4 | Number cycles in sequence |

Temperature taken	R		(R) Rectally
	V		(V) Vaginally
	O	X	(O) Orally

Earliest first higher temperature reading in the previous cycles

1 5

Minus 8 7

This information is used to identify the infertile time at the beginning of the cycle

Earliest first higher temperature reading in this cycle 1 4

Do you intend to become pregnant in the next cycle?

yes

no X

undecided

❂ Malteser
...weil Nähe zählt.

Figure 2: The cycle chart with explanation of entries

Observing cervical mucus and recording on the cycle chart

Making cervical mucus observations requires you to feel, see, and touch your cervical mucus throughout the day and evening. At the end of the day, enter your description of the best cervical mucus quality observed on the rows marked "Mucus." (cf. Manual *Natural & Safe: The Handbook*).

The cervical mucus observations for each day are summarized with a corresponding abbreviation and can be entered on or above the 37 °C line on the cycle chart. (Table 1 and Figure 3).

Daily cervical mucus observations should begin toward the end of menstruation.

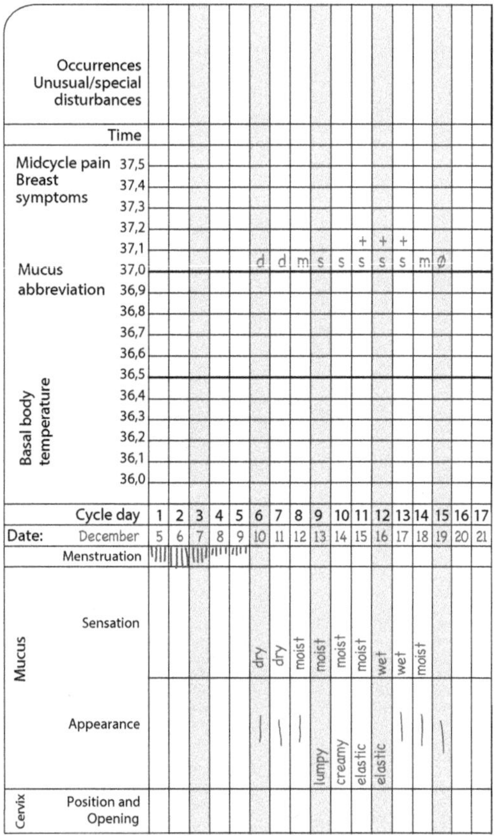

Figure 3: Enter the cervical mucus observations on the cycle chart.

Table 1: Cervical mucus classifications, observations and abbreviations

Feel/Touch		Appearance	Code
dry, rough, itching, unpleasant feeling	and	no visible mucus, no cervical mucus at the vaginal opening	▷ d
no mucus felt, no moistness, presence of mucus not sensed at the vaginal opening	and	no visible mucus, no cervical mucus at the vaginal opening	▷ ø
moist	but	no visible mucus, no cervical mucus at the vaginal opening	▷ m
moist but presence of mucus not sensed	and	thick, whitish, opaque, creamy, lumpy, yellowish, sticky, milky, non-elastic or tough	▷ S
moist, but presence of mucus not sensed	and	translucent, transparent, translucent sheen like raw egg white (translucent with white streaks), elastic or stretchy, can be stretched into strands, so liquid that it "runs like water", reddish, red-brown, yellowish-red	+ ▷ S
wet, slimy, slippery, lubricating, like oil, smooth	and/ or	translucent, transparent, translucent sheen like raw egg white (translucent with white streaks), elastic or stretchy, can be stretched into strands, so liquid that it "runs like water", reddish, red-brown, yellowish-red	+ ▷ S

Observing basal body temperature and recording on the cycle chart

First morning body temperature (basal body temperature) has two temperature phases during a cycle. Before ovulation, in the follicular phase, basal body temperature is slightly lower. After ovulation, it increases by a few tenths of a °C (cf. Manual *Natural & Safe: The Handbook*).

How to measure your temperature

- Immediately after waking and before getting out of bed
- After at least one hour of rest or sleep
- Ideally every day
- By using an analog basal body thermometer or a calibrated digital thermometer displaying two decimal points
- Always use the same method: orally, rectally, or vaginally (hold for 3 minutes); never under the arm

What can disturb or affect temperature?

- Changing thermometer mid-cycle
- Change in the measuring method
- Different measuring times
- Change in the environment (traveling, holiday, vacations, change in climate)
- Stress, mental strain, excitement
- Unaccustomed alcohol consumption, partying late into the night
- Late meal in the evening
- Unusually late bedtime
- Not sleeping long enough or broken sleep
- Shift work
- Illnesses and ailments
- Some medications

All disturbances are noted on the row marked "Occurrences, Unusual/special disturbances."

Special features of digital thermometers

- Thermometer should have a valid calibration stamp
- Continue measuring for three minutes after the beep
- Use a digital thermometer that measures to two decimal points
- Round the value up or down to half a tenth of a °C
- If the temperature curve is unclear, or if in doubt, use a second thermometer as a comparison during the cycle

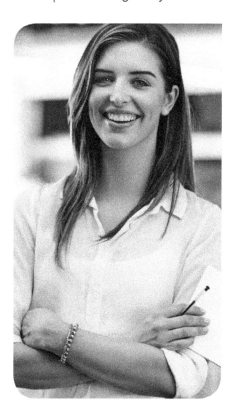

Figure 4: Enter the temperature values

		Cycle day	1	2	3	4	5	6	7	8	9	10	11	12	13	14	15	16	17	18	19	20	21	22	23	24	25	26	27	28	29	30	31	32	33	34	35	36	37	38	39	40

Occurrences
Unusual/special
disturbances

Time

Midcycle pain
Breast symptoms

Mucus abbreviation

Basal body temperature

37,5
37,4
37,3
37,2
37,1
37,0
36,9
36,8
36,7
36,6
36,5
36,4
36,3
36,2
36,1
36,0

Date:

Menstruation

Mucus — Sensation

Mucus — Appearance

Cervix — Position and opening

Cervix — Firmness

Intercourse

Fertile Days

Arbeitsgruppe NFP ©

Recording cervical mucus observations

» **Susanne P., who does not wish to become pregnant this cycle, has decided to learn Sensiplan; this is the first cycle she is recording.**

Enter the following in the cycle chart: all important information, cervical mucus observations, and corresponding abbreviations on the 37 °C line (Solution in Training 2).

1st cycle day: The cycle begins on the first day of menstruation, which is October 11th; her bleeding is heavy.

2nd cycle day: Menstrual bleeding is quite heavy

3rd and 4th cycle days: Menstrual bleeding is lighter

5th cycle day: Susanne P. is not bleeding anymore. She feels that her vagina is dry and she does not notice cervical mucus.

6th cycle day: She does not feel anything at her vagina, does not feel "moist," and cannot see any cervical mucus.

7th cycle day: Susanne P. feels moist a few times, but cannot see any cervical mucus.

8th and 9th cycle days: She feels moist again and notices white, lumpy cervical mucus that is not elastic.

10th cycle day: During the day she notices white cervical mucus and feels moist. In the evening the cervical mucus is transparent and elastic.

11th cycle day: During the day she has the feeling that the toilet paper easily glides across her vagina. Her vagina feels wet, and she notices that her cervical mucus can form threads that are several centimeters long.

12th and 13th cycle days: Susanne P. feels that her vagina is completely wet, and on day 13 she even has the feeling that it is running like water.

14th cycle day: She feels moist all day and notices that she has elastic cervical mucus.

15th cycle day: She still feels moist; however, her cervical mucus looks creamy again.

16th cycle day: Her vaginal area still feels moist, but Susanne P. cannot see any more cervical mucus.

17th and 18th cycle days: She cannot feel or see any more cervical mucus.

Basal body temperature chart

Row	1	2	3	4	5	6	7	8	9	10	11	12	13	14	15	16	17	18	19	20	21	22	23
Temp marker (37,1)								+	+	+	+	+											
Mucus abbreviation (37,0)			d	Ø	m	S	S	S	S	S	S	S	S	m	Ø	Ø							

Occurrences / Unusual/special disturbances — (blank)

Time — (blank)

Midcycle pain / Breast symptoms — (blank)

Basal body temperature scale: 37,5 · 37,4 · 37,3 · 37,2 · 37,1 · 37,0 · 36,9 · 36,8 · 36,7 · 36,6 · 36,5 · 36,4 · 36,3 · 36,2 · 36,1 · 36,0

Cycle day	1	2	3	4	5	6	7	8	9	10	11	12	13	14	15	16	17	18	19	20	21	22	23	24	25	26	27	28	29	30	31	32	33	34	35	36	37	38	39	40
Date: October	11	12	13	14	15	16	17	18	19	20	21	22	23	24	25	26	27	28	29	30	31	11/1	2	3	4	5	6	7	8	9	10	11	12	13	14	15	16	17	18	19

Menstruation: markings on cycle days 1–6

Mucus

	1	2	3	4	5	6	7	8	9	10	11	12	13	14	15	16	17
Sensation				dry	nothing	moist	moist	moist	moist	wet	wet	wet	moist	moist	moist	nothing	nothing
Appearance							white/lumpy	white/lumpy	transparent/elastic	forms threads		runs like water	elastic	creamy			

Cervix

Position and opening — (blank)

Firmness — (blank)

Intercourse — (blank)

Fertile Days — (blank)

Arbeitsgruppe NFP ©

Recording temperature

» **Susanne P. measures her basal body temperature every morning between 6 and 7 o'clock with an analog thermometer. She measures her temperatures rectally.**

Enter all important observations on the cycle chart. The solution for training 1 is already entered here.

1st cycle day: Her temperature is between the lines of 36.6 and 36.7.

2nd cycle day: Her temperature is 36.7.

3rd cycle day: She forgets to measure.

4th cycle day: The thermometer reads 36.6.

5th cycle day: Susanne P. does not measure until 10 o'clock; also, she had alcohol the evening before at a party. The thermometer reads 36.9.

6th cycle day: Her temperature when she wakes up is 36.6.

7th cycle day: Her temperature when she wakes up is 36.6.

8th and 9th cycle days: Susanne P. reads the thermometer at 36.5.

10th cycle day: Her temperature is between the lines of 36.5 and 36.6.

11th cycle day: Susanne P's temperature when she wakes up is 36.7.

12th cycle days: Her temperature goes back down to 36.5.

13th cycle day: The thermometer reads 36.6.

14th and 15th cycle days: Her temperature is 36.8 on both days.

16th cycle day: Susanne P. measures 36.85.

17th cycle days: Her temperature is 36.9.

18th cycle day: Susanne P. measures 36.85 again.

Because Susanne P. does not yet know how to identify the infertile phase at the beginning of the cycle, and she has no information from her past cycles, in the 1st cycle, she has to assume that she is fertile starting on cycle day 1.

She will enter "F" on the row marked "Fertile Days" each day until she learns to identify the beginning of the infertile time after ovulation using the Sensiplan rules.

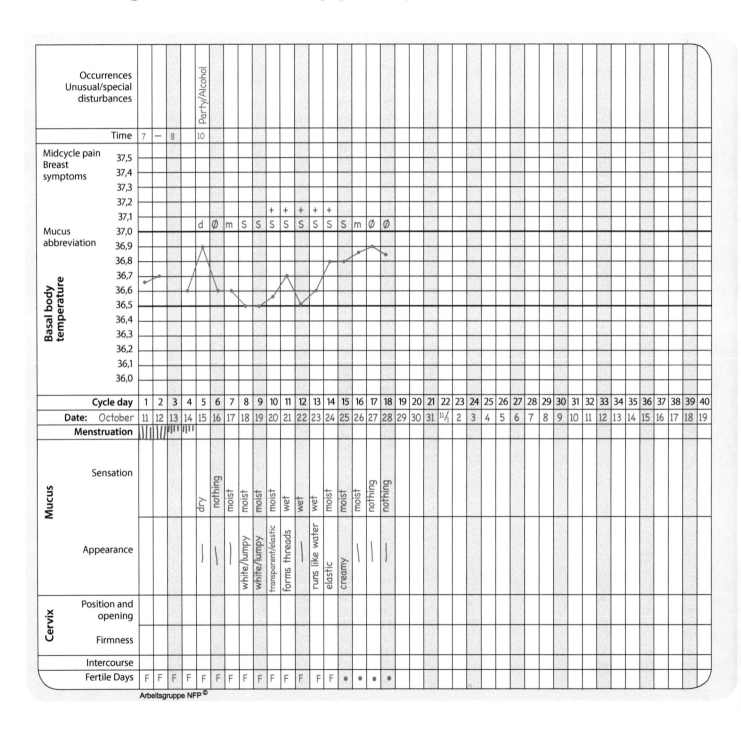

Arbeitsgruppe NFP ©

®

Cycle-no* | 1 |

Temperature taken R [X]
V [ ]
O [ ]

Earliest first higher
temperature reading
in the previous cycles

[|]

Minus 8   [|]

Earliest first higher
temperature
reading in
this cycle   [|]

Do you intend to
become pregnant
in the next cycle?

yes [ ]
no [X]
undecided [ ]

✶ **Malteser**
...weil Nähe zählt.

Enter the temperature

» Susanne P. recorded all her measured temperature values. Since she did not measure on the 3rd day of her cycle, the readings from the 2nd and 4th day of the cycle are not connected.

		Cycle day values →		

Occurrences Unusual/special disturbances

Time

Midcycle pain / Breast symptoms

Mucus abbreviation

Basal body temperature — scale: 37,5 · 37,4 · 37,3 · 37,2 · 37,1 · 37,0 · 36,9 · 36,8 · 36,7 · 36,6 · 36,5 · 36,4 · 36,3 · 36,2 · 36,1 · 36,0

Cycle day	1	2	3	4	5	6	7	8	9	10	11	12	13	14	15	16	17	18	19	20	21	22	23	24	25	26	27	28	29	30	31	32	33	34	35	36	37	38	39	40
Date: December	12	13	14	15	16	17	18	19	20	21	22	23	24	25	26	27	28	29	30	31	1/1	2	3	4	5	6	7	8	9	10	11	12	13	14	15	16	17	18	19	20
Menstruation	‖	‖	‖	‖	‖	‖	‖																						‖	‖	‖	‖								
Mucus – Sensation						moist	moist	moist	moist	moist	moist	moist	moist	moist	wet	moist	nothing	nothing																						
Mucus – Appearance						(mark)	(mark)	(mark)	thick	thick	sticky	stretchy	stretchy	translucent	liquid	thick	(mark)	(mark)																						
Cervix – Position and opening																																								
Cervix – Firmness																																								
Intercourse																																								
Fertile Days																																								

37,00	37,00
36,99	
36,98	
36,97	
36,96	
36,95	36,95
36,94	
36,93	
36,92	
36,91	
36,90	36,90
36,89	
36,88	
36,87	
36,86	
36,85	36,85
36,84	
36,83	
36,82	
36,81	
36,80	36,80
36,79	
36,78	
36,77	
36,76	
36,75	36,75
36,74	
36,73	
36,72	
36,71	
36,70	36,70
36,69	
36,68	
36,67	
36,66	
36,65	36,65
36,64	
36,63	
36,62	
36,61	
36,60	36,60
36,59	
36,58	
36,57	
36,56	
36,55	36,55
36,54	
36,53	
36,52	
36,51	
36,50	36,50
36,49	
36,48	
36,47	
36,46	
36,45	36,45
36,44	
36,43	
36,42	
36,41	
36,40	36,40
36,39	
36,38	
36,37	
36,36	
36,35	36,35
36,34	
36,33	
36,32	
36,31	
36,30	36,30
36,29	
36,28	
36,27	
36,26	
36,25	36,25
36,24	
36,23	
36,22	
36,21	
36,20	36,20
36,19	
36,18	
36,17	
36,16	
36,15	36,15
36,14	
36,13	
36,12	
36,11	
36,10	36,10
36,09	
36,08	
36,07	
36,06	
36,05	36,05
36,04	
36,03	
36,02	
36,01	
36,00	36,00

Sidebar form

SENSIPLAN ®

Cycle-no* | 3 |

Temperature taken R | |
V | |
O | |

Earliest first higher temperature reading in the previous cycles | | |

Minus 8 | | |

Earliest first higher temperature reading in this cycle | | |

Do you intend to become pregnant in the next cycle?

yes | |
no | |
undecided | |

Malteser
...weil Nähe zählt.

Recording temperature and cervical mucus observations

» Susanne P. recorded all her measured temperature values. Since she did not measure on the 3rd day of her cycle, the readings from the 2nd and 4th day of the cycle are not connected.

First, record the cervical mucus abbreviations on or above the 37 °C line on the cycle chart. Then record the following temperatures. Round the temperature values up or down to half a tenth of a °C (cf. Table 2 and manual *Natural & Safe: The Handbook*).

On **day 4** of the cycle the digital temperature reading is 36.44.
On **day 5** of the cycle the digital temperature reading is 36.48.
On **day 6** of the cycle the digital temperature reading is 36.38.
On **day 7** of the cycle the digital temperature reading is 36.56.
On **day 8** of the cycle the digital temperature reading is 36.59.
On **day 9** of the cycle the digital temperature reading is 36.42.
On **day 10** of the cycle the digital temperature reading is 36.34.
On **day 11** of the cycle the digital temperature reading is 36.49.
On **day 12** of the cycle the digital temperature reading is 36.40.
On **day 13** of the cycle the digital temperature reading is 36.32.
On **day 14** of the cycle the digital temperature reading is 36.45.
On **day 15** of the cycle the digital temperature reading is 36.33.
On **day 16** of the cycle the digital temperature reading is 36.55.
On **day 17** of the cycle the digital temperature reading is 36.66.
On **day 18** of the cycle the digital temperature reading is 36.74

Table. 2: Rounding off with a digital thermometer

Refer to the table at left and the examples below to determine how to round (up or down) individual temperatures taken.

36.50 = 36.50	36.51 = 36.50	36.52 = 36.50
36.53 = 36.55	36.54 = 36.55	36.55 = 36.55
36.56 = 36.55	36.57 = 36.55	
36.58 = 36.60	36.59 = 36.60	36.60 = 36.60

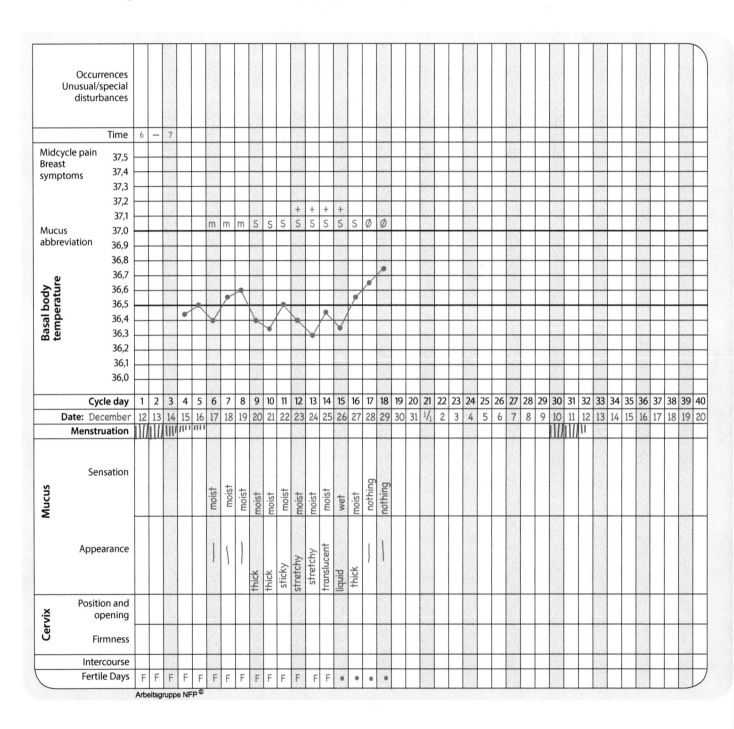

		Cycle day	1	2	3	4	5	6	7	8	9	10	11	12	13	14	15	16	17	18	19	20	21	22	23	24	25	26	27	28	29	30	31	32	33	34	35	36	37	38	39	40

Time: 6 — 7

Mucus abbreviation: m m m S S S S S S S S Ø Ø (cycle days 6–18)

Date: December 12 13 14 15 16 17 18 19 20 21 22 23 24 25 26 27 28 29 30 31 1/1 2 3 4 5 6 7 8 9 10 11 12 13 14 15 16 17 18 19 20

Mucus – Sensation: moist, moist, moist, moist, moist, moist, moist, moist, moist, wet, moist, nothing, nothing

Mucus – Appearance: thick, thick, sticky, stretchy, stretchy, translucent, liquid, thick

Fertile Days: F F F F F F F F F F F F F F F F • • • •

Arbeitsgruppe NFP ©

®

Cycle-no*   [ ] 3

Temperature taken   R [X]

V [ ]

O [ ]

Earliest first higher
temperature reading
in the previous cycles

[|]

Minus 8   [|]

Earliest first higher
temperature
reading in
this cycle

[|]

Do you intend to
become pregnant
in the next cycle?

yes [ ]

no [ ]

undecided [ ]

�֍ **Malteser**
...weil Nähe zählt.

Recording temperature and cervical mucus observations

» In the third cycle, Susanne P. measured her temperature using a digital thermometer. She recorded her temperature values and cervical mucus abbreviations on the cycle chart shown at left.

Occurrences Unusual/special disturbances

Time

Midcycle pain
Breast symptoms

Mucus abbreviation

Basal body temperature

Temperature
37,5
37,4
37,3
37,2
37,1
37,0
36,9
36,8
36,7
36,6
36,5
36,4
36,3
36,2
36,1
36,0

Cycle day	1	2	3	4	5	6	7	8	9	10	11	12	13	14	15	16	17	18	19	20	21	22	23	24	25	26	27	28	29	30	31	32	33	34	35	36	37	38	39	40
Date: January	25	26	27	28	29	30	31	²/₁	2	3	4	5	6	7	8	9	10	11	12	13	14	15	16	17	18	19	20	21	22	23	24	25	26	27	28	³/₁	2	3	4	5
Menstruation																																								

Mucus

Sensation: nothing, nothing, nothing, moist, moist, wet, wet, wet, moist, moist, dry, ... moist, ... moist, wet

Appearance: yellowish, yellowish, whitish, lumpy, lumpy, stretchy, ... yellowish, ... transparent

Cervix

Position and opening

Firmness

Intercourse

Fertile Days

Arbeitsgruppe NFP ©

Cervical mucus abbreviations

» Julia T., a 17-year-old student, would like to learn more about her body. Although she is making cervical mucus observations, she reports having difficulty choosing the correct cervical mucus abbreviations.

Enter the abbreviations on or above the 37 °C line.

---

sensiplan ®

Cycle-no* 3

Temperature taken R

V

O

Earliest first higher temperature reading in the previous cycles

Minus 8

Earliest first higher temperature reading in this cycle

Do you intend to become pregnant in the next cycle?

yes

no

undecided

✠ **Malteser**

...weil Nähe zählt.

Occurrences Unusual/special disturbances			

Time

Midcycle pain / Breast symptoms

Mucus abbreviation / **Basal body temperature**

Temp (°C)	
37,5	
37,4	
37,3	
37,2	
37,1	+ + + (days 12,13,14); + (day 28)
37,0	Mucus abbreviations: Ø Ø S S S S S S S m d Ø Ø Ø Ø Ø S Ø Ø Ø m S
36,9	
36,8	
36,7	
36,6	
36,5	
36,4	
36,3	
36,2	
36,1	
36,0	

Cycle day	1	2	3	4	5	6	7	8	9	10	11	12	13	14	15	16	17	18	19	20	21	22	23	24	25	26	27	28	29	30	31	32	33	34	35	36	37	38	39	40
Date: January	25	26	27	28	29	30	31	2/1	2	3	4	5	6	7	8	9	10	11	12	13	14	15	16	17	18	19	20	21	22	23	24	25	26	27	28	3/1	2	3	4	5
Menstruation	‖	‖	‖	‖	‖	‖																						‖												

Mucus

Sensation	day 7: nothing; 8: nothing; 9: nothing; 10: moist; 11: moist; 12: wet; 13: wet; 14: wet; 15: moist; 16: moist; 17: dry; 18: |; 19: |; 20: |; 21: |; 23: moist; 25: |; 26: |; 27: moist; 28: wet
Appearance	day 7: |; 8: |; 9: yellowish; 10: yellowish; 11: whitish; 12: lumpy; 13: stretchy; 14: |; 15: yellowish; 16: |; 17: |; 18: |; 19: |; 20: |; 23: yellowish; 25: |; 26: |; 27: |; 28: transparent

Cervix

Position and opening	
Firmness	

Intercourse	
Fertile Days	

Arbeitsgruppe NFP ©

®

Cycle-no* | 3

Temperature taken
R ☐
V ☐
O ☐

Earliest first higher
temperature reading
in the previous cycles
☐☐

Minus 8 ☐☐

Earliest first higher
temperature
reading in
this cycle
☐☐

Do you intend to
become pregnant
in the next cycle?

yes ☐
no ☐
undecided ☐

✠ **Malteser**
...weil Nähe zählt.

Cervical mucus abbreviations

» Using the cervical mucus abbreviation table, Julia T. entered the cervical mucus abbreviations on her cycle chart.

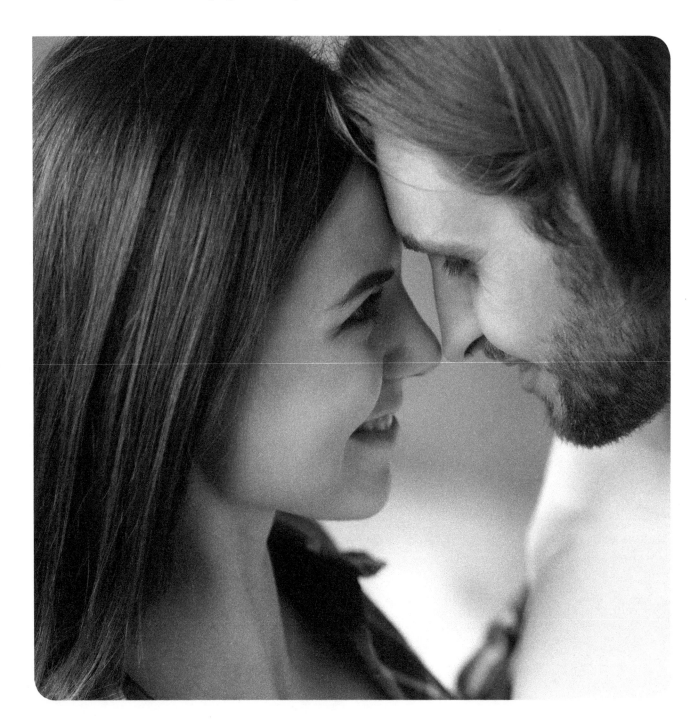

Measuring temperature

Quiz

Check the corresponding box to indicate if the statement is true or false.	TRUE	FALSE
Basal body temperature should be measured in the morning after getting out of bed.		
An analog thermometer can be used to measure basal body temperature.		
Measuring at different times of the day will always affect the temperature measurement.		
Times that differ from the usual measuring time must be recorded on the cycle chart.		
If you wake up during the night, you must sleep or rest for at least an hour before measuring your temperature.		
Changing your thermometer midway through the cycle will not affect the temperature evaluation.		
Temperature can be measured in the anus (rectally), in the vagina (vaginally) or in the mouth (orally).		
The same measuring technique should be used throughout a cycle and noted on the cycle chart.		
Measuring your temperature rectally takes 10 minutes.		
You can measure at any time of the morning without affecting the temperature value.		
Measuring your temperature after being awake for a few hours will not impact your interpretation of the chart.		
Changes to your usual habits such as stress, travel, or illness, should be recorded on the cycle chart in the row marked "Occurrences, unusual/special disturbances."		
If you measure your temperature using a digital thermometer, the exact value shown should be recorded on the cycle chart.		
Events that may affect your temperature measurement should be entered on the cycle chart on the day they affect.		

Temperature Quiz Solution

Check the corresponding box to indicate if the statement is true or false.	TRUE	FALSE
Basal body temperature should be measured in the morning after getting out of bed.		X
An analog thermometer can be used to measure basal body temperature.	X	
Measuring at different times of the day will always affect the temperature measurement.		X
Times that differ from the usual measuring time must be recorded on the cycle chart.	X	
If you wake up during the night, you must sleep or rest for at least an hour before measuring your temperature.	X	
Changing your thermometer midway through the cycle will not affect the temperature evaluation.		X
Temperature can be measured in the anus (rectally), in the vagina (vaginally), or in the mouth (orally).	X	
The same measuring technique should be used throughout a cycle and noted on the cycle chart.	X	
Measuring your temperature rectally takes 10 minutes.		X
You can measure at any time of the morning without affecting the temperature value.		X
Measuring your temperature after being awake for a few hours will not impact your interpretation of the chart.		X
Changes to your usual habits such as stress, travel, or illness, should be recorded on the cycle chart in the row marked "Occurrences, unusual/special disturbances."	X	
If you measure your temperature using a digital thermometer, the exact value shown should be recorded on the cycle chart.		X
Events that may affect your temperature measurement should be entered on the cycle chart on the day they affect.	X	

(For reasons and detailed explanation, please see manual *Natural & Safe: The Handbook*)

Observing the cervix and other signs, and recording on the cycle chart

Like cervical mucus and temperature, the cervix also undergoes changes throughout the cycle. Changes of the cervix can be monitored as an alternative to cervical mucus observations. It is recommended that you do not use this method until you have mastered making and recording cervical mucus observations. In our experience, this typically takes at least two observation cycles.

How is the cervix examined?
- Once a day
- In the same position and always with the same finger
- In a slightly stooped position

What is assessed?
- The width of the opening of the cervix (closed, partially open, completely open)
- The position (lower/higher)
- The firmness (hard or soft)

Other body signs
Other body signs can contribute to a woman understanding her fertility. These signs may include breast tenderness, mid-cycle pain, spotting, skin symptoms, water retention (edema), weight fluctuations, physical performance changes, or an increase or decrease in libido. These signs cannot be evaluated using a hard and fast rule, however, they may give women additional valuable information.

Breast symptoms (B) and mid-cycle pain (M) should be noted on the assigned lines on the cycle chart. Other symptoms are recorded on the row marked "Occurrences, unusual/special disturbances."

Figure 5: Make and record observations of the cervix and other signs

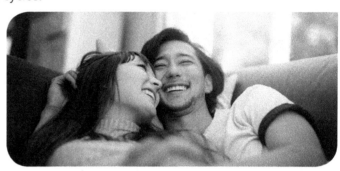

	Cycle day	1	2	3	4	5	6	7	8	9	10	11	12	13	14	15	16	17	18	19	20	21	22	23	24	25	26	27	28	29	30	31	32	33	34	35	36	37	38	39	40
Occurrences Unusual/special disturbances																Edema	Edema																									
Midcycle pain / Breast symptoms / Mucus abbreviation	Time													M	M		B	B	B																						
Cervix — Position and Opening							•	•	•	•	•	○	○	○	Ⓞ	○	○	○	•	•	•	•	•	•																	
Cervix — Firmness							hard	hard	hard	hard	softer	soft	soft	soft	soft	softer	harder	hard	hard	hard	hard	hard																			
Date: June		3	4	5	6	7	8	9	10	11	12	13	14	15	16	17	18	19	20	21	22	23	24	25																	

Basal body temperature scale: 37,5 / 37,4 / 37,3 / 37,2 / 37,1 / 37,0 / 36,9 / 36,8 / 36,7 / 36,6 / 36,5 / 36,4 / 36,3 / 36,2 / 36,1 / 36,0

Rows: Menstruation; Mucus — Sensation, Appearance; Cervix — Position and Opening, Firmness; Intercourse; Fertile Days

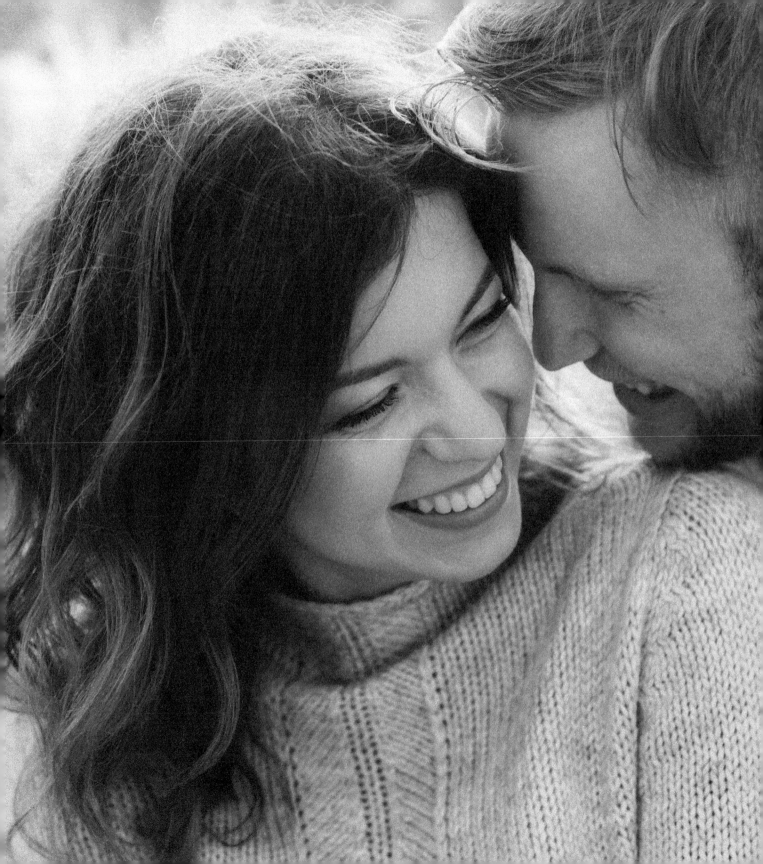

Chapter 2

The infertile time after ovulation

The fertile and infertile times are identified using signs of fertility. This chapter explains how the infertile time after ovulation can be identified using a double check with cervical mucus and basal body temperature.

Identifying the infertile time after ovulation

For a Sensiplan beginner, identifying the infertile time after ovulation is the easiest part of learning Sensiplan; this is done using cervical mucus and temperature recordings. The shift of cervical mucus quality and the increase in basal body temperature are used to mark the end of the fertile time, using the double check principle.

Evaluating cervical mucus observations

Rule: Shift of the cervical mucus sign

The cervical mucus shift is the last day of your best quality cervical mucus before it shifts to a lower quality. Determining the day of this shift (Peak day) can only be done after it has happened. On the chart below, the letter "P" shows the Peak day, or the last day of the best quality cervical mucus before the shift to a lower quality.

How is the cervical mucus sign evaluated?

First, determine the last day of your best quality cervical mucus before it shifts to a lower quality and mark it with a "P" above the cervical mucus abbreviation. Then mark the next three days as 1 - 2 - 3 (cf. *Natural & Safe: The Handbook*). (Figure 6)

Evaluating cervix observations

Rule: Cervix

If you choose to use the cervix sign instead of the cervical mucus sign, the infertile time after ovulation begins on the evening of the third day with a closed and hard cervix, using a double check with temperature measurements (cf. *Natural & Safe: The Handbook*) (Figure 7)

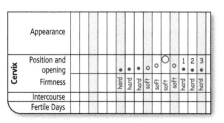

Figure 7: Evaluating the position of the cervix

Evaluating temperature measurements

Rule: Temperature shift

A temperature shift can be confirmed when three consecutive readings are all higher than the six previous readings, and the 3rd higher reading is at least 2 boxes (2/10°C) above the previous six lower-temperature readings. (Figure 8)

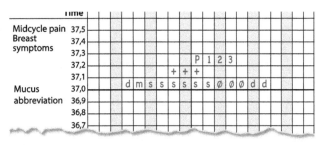
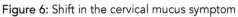

Figure 6: Shift in the cervical mucus symptom

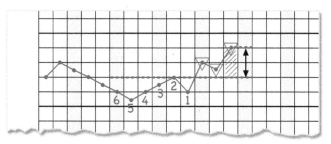

Figure 8: Evaluation of the temperature shift

How is it done?

Rule: Each day your new temperature measurement is compared with the temperature measurements from the six previous days. Temperature measurements where there have been "disturbances" are put in brackets and are not taken into account. Look for the temperature that is higher than any of the previous six temperature measurements. A cover line is drawn at the level of the highest of these six previous lower values. The next day's temperature must be higher than the cover line.

If the criteria for the rule have been met and the third higher measurement is 2/10 °C above the cover line, draw a triangle around the three higher readings on the cycle chart. The temperature evaluation is now complete (cf. *Natural & Safe: The Handbook*).

First exception to the rule on temperature:

If the 3rd temperature measurement is not 2/10 °C higher than the cover line, a 4th temperature measurement must be used. This also must be higher than the cover line, but it does not necessarily have to be 2/10°C higher. (Figure 9)

Second exception to the rule on temperature:

Out of three required higher temperature measurements, one measurement may fall down to or below the cover line. This value must not be taken into account and is therefore not triangled. The third value, however, must be at least 2/10 °C (2 boxes) above the cover line. (Figure 10)

The first and second exceptions to the rule cannot be used together in the same cycle.

Identifying the infertile time after ovulation -

Rule: Double check of cervical mucus and temperature

The infertile time after ovulation begins on the evening of the 3rd day after the cervical mucus shift or the evening of the 3rd higher temperature measurement, whichever comes last (cf. *Natural & Safe: The Handbook*).

The beginning of the infertile time after ovulation is marked with an F/ in the row marked "Fertile Days."

Another option

Rule: Double check of cervix position and temperature

The infertile time after ovulation begins on the evening of the 3rd day with a closed and hard cervix, or the evening of the 3rd higher temperature measurement, whichever comes last (cf. *Natural & Safe: The Handbook*).

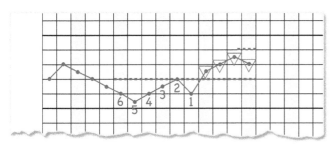

Figure 9: First exception to the rule

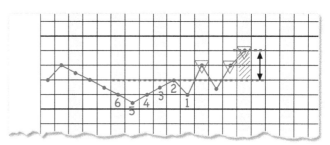

Figure 10: Second exception to the rule

				+	+					
d	d	d	m	S	S	S	S	S	d	d	d

						+	+			
S	S	S	S	S	S	S	S	m	S	m	m	m

d	d	m	m	S	S	d	d	d	d	d	d	d

				+	+		+			
Ø	Ø	m	S	S	S	S	S	S	m	m	d	d

			+							
d	d	m	S	S	S	S	S	m	m	Ø	Ø	Ø

					+	+	+			
Ø	Ø	Ø	m	m	S	S	S	S	S	S	S	Ø

m	m	m	m	m	m	S	m	m	m	m	Ø	Ø	Ø

d	d	Ø	Ø	Ø	m	m	m	Ø	Ø	Ø	d	d

Identifying the cervical mucus shift

Every woman has her own individual cervical mucus pattern. While most women notice S+ quality cervical mucus in each cycle, some rarely or never observe this type of cervical mucus. These women can still learn how to determine the shift in their cervical mucus. At left, are some examples.

Evaluate the cervical mucus observations by marking the shift with a "P" above the abbreviation and numbering the next three days (P -1 -2 -3).

Training 6 - Solution   The infertile time after ovulation

Chart 1:

							P	1	2	3			
						+	+						
d	d	d	m	S	S	S	S	S	d	d	d	d	

Chart 2:

								P	1	2	3		
							+	+					
S	S	S	S	S	S	S	S	m	S	m	m	m	

Chart 3:

					P	1	2	3					
d	d	m	m	S	S	d	d	d	d	d	d	d	

Chart 4:

						P	1	P	1	2	3		
					+	+		+					
Ø	Ø	m	S	S	S	S	S	S	m	m	d	d	

Chart 5:

				P	1	2	3					
			+									
d	d	m	S	S	S	S	S	m	m	Ø	Ø	Ø

Chart 6:

							P	1	2	3		
					+	+	+					
Ø	Ø	Ø	m	m	S	S	S	S	S	S	S	Ø

Chart 7:

						P	1	2	3			
m	m	m	m	m	m	S	m	m	m	m	Ø	Ø	Ø

Chart 8:

						P	1	2	3			
d	d	Ø	Ø	Ø	m	m	m	Ø	Ø	Ø	d	d

Identifying the cervical mucus shift

The examples show that even with lower quality cervical mucus the shift in the cervical mucus symptom can be reliably identified.

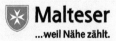

	Cycle day	1	2	3	4	5	6	7	8	9	10	11	12	13	14	15	16	17	18	19	20	21	22	23	24	25	26	27	28	29	30	31	32	33	34	35	36	37	38	39	40
	Date: November	18	19	20	21	22	23	24	25	26	27	28	29	30	12/1	2	3	4	5	6	7	8	9	10	11	12	13	14	15	16	17	18	19	20	21	22	23	24	25	26	27

Time row: 6³⁰, 6³⁰, 7, 6³⁰, 6³⁰, 7, 7, 10 (late to bed), 7, 7, 6³⁰, 6³⁰, 6³⁰, 7, 7, 7, 7, 6³⁰, 6³⁰, 7, 7, 6³⁰, 6³⁰, 7, 7, 6³⁰, 6³⁰, 7, 7, 6³⁰, 7

Occurrences / Unusual/special disturbances: late to bed (day 8)

Basal body temperature (°C): scale 36,0 – 37,5

Menstruation: cycle days 1–5 (Nov 18–22) and days 32–34 (Nov 19–21)

Mucus – Sensation: dry (day 6), dry (day 7), moist (day 8), moist (day 9), moist (day 10), moist (day 11), wet (day 12), wet (day 13), wet (day 14), moist (day 15)

Mucus – Appearance: lumpy (day 8), lumpy (day 9), whitish (day 10), stretchy (day 11), stretchy (day 12), translucent (day 13), thick (day 14), sticky (day 15)

Cervix – Position and opening: (blank)

Cervix – Firmness: (blank)

Intercourse: X (day 22), X (day 24)

Fertile Days: (blank)

Arbeitsgruppe NFP ©

Identifying the infertile time after ovulation

Cycle-no*		1

Temperature taken	R	X
	V	
	O	

Earliest first higher temperature reading in the previous cycles

Minus 8

Earliest first higher temperature reading in this cycle

Do you intend to become pregnant in the next cycle?

yes	
no	X
undecided	

Malteser
...weil Nähe zählt.

» **Michaela S. is a 23-year-old businesswoman who recently completed her first cycle chart using Sensiplan.**

1. Enter the cervical mucus abbreviations and identify the shift in the cervical mucus sign.

2. Are there any disturbances or special circumstances?

3. Identify the earliest first higher temperature reading and enter this in the column on the right.

4. Determine the beginning of the infertile time after ovulation and mark all fertile days with an "F."

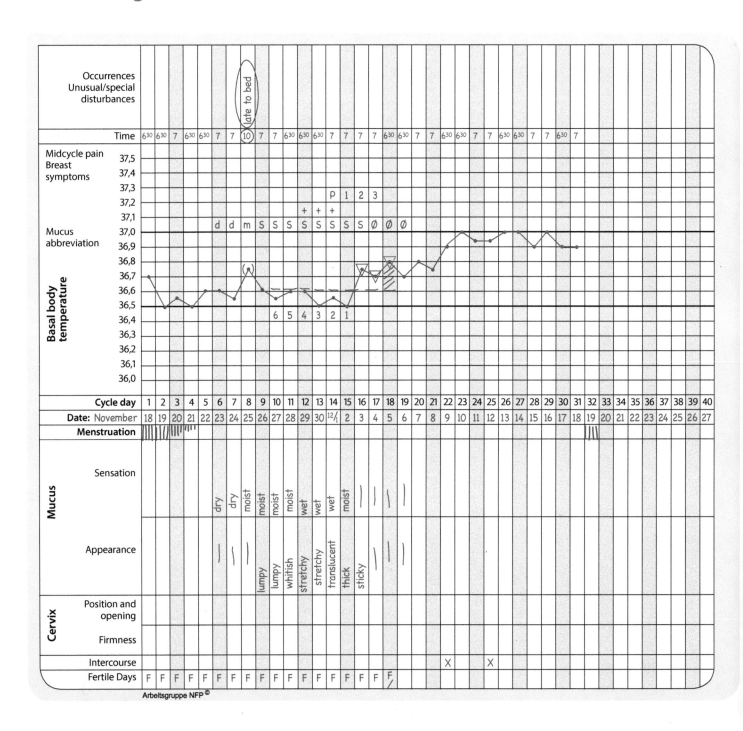

Arbeitsgruppe NFP ©

Cycle-no* | | 1

®

**Temperature
taken** R [X]

V [ ]

O [ ]

Earliest first higher
temperature reading
in the previous cycles

[|]

Minus 8 [|]

Earliest first higher
temperature
reading in [1|6]
this cycle

Do you intend to
become pregnant
in the next cycle?

yes [ ]

no [X]

undecided [ ]

✠ Malteser
...weil Nähe zählt.

Identifying the infertile time after ovulation

1. The shift of the cervical mucus sign is on cycle day 14.

2. The temperature measurement on cycle day 8 is a disturbance and is put in brackets. The disturbance is noted because "late to bed" and a later-than-usual temperature measurement were recorded.

3. The earliest first higher temperature reading is on cycle day 16.

4. The infertile time after ovulation begins on the evening of cycle day 18 and is marked by "F/."

Note:
- Since Michaela S. is observing her first cycle using Sensiplan, fertility is assumed starting Cycle Day 1.

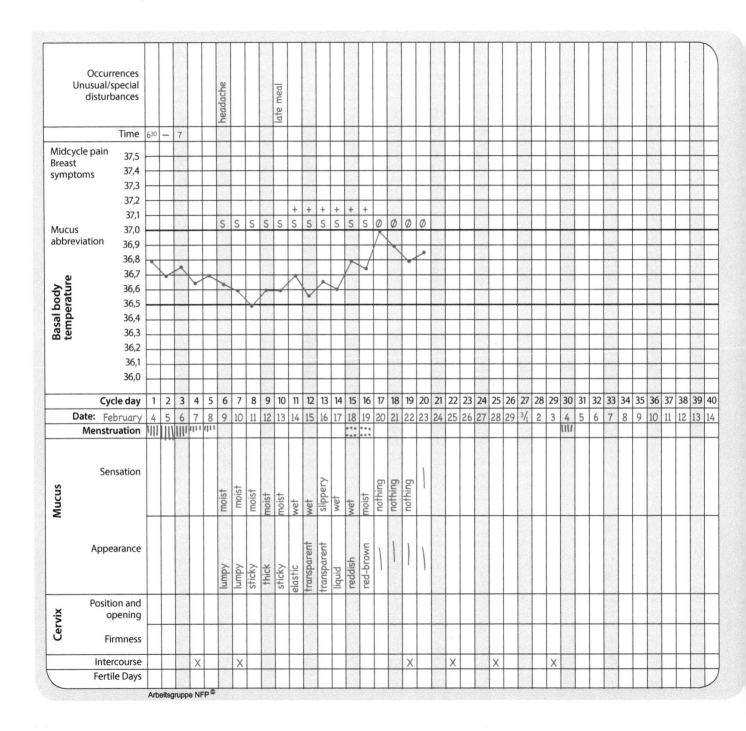

Occurrences Unusual/special disturbances: headache (day 6), late meal (day 9)

Time: 6³⁰ — 7

Midcycle pain / Breast symptoms / Mucus abbreviation

Temperature scale: 37,5 / 37,4 / 37,3 / 37,2 / 37,1 / 37,0 / 36,9 / 36,8 / 36,7 / 36,6 / 36,5 / 36,4 / 36,3 / 36,2 / 36,1 / 36,0

Mucus abbreviation row: S S S S S S S S S S S S Ø Ø Ø Ø

"+" marks at cycle days 11–16 (37,1 line)

Cycle day	1	2	3	4	5	6	7	8	9	10	11	12	13	14	15	16	17	18	19	20	21	22	23	24	25	26	27	28	29	30	31	32	33	34	35	36	37	38	39	40
Date: February	4	5	6	7	8	9	10	11	12	13	14	15	16	17	18	19	20	21	22	23	24	25	26	27	28	29	³/₁	2	3	4	5	6	7	8	9	10	11	12	13	14

Menstruation: marks on days 1–5 and days 18–19, and around day 30

Mucus — Sensation: moist (6), moist (7), moist (8), moist (9), moist (10), wet (11), wet (12), slippery (13), wet (14), wet (15), moist (16), nothing (17), nothing (18), nothing (19), | (20)

Mucus — Appearance: lumpy (6), lumpy (7), sticky (8), thick (9), sticky (10), elastic (11), transparent (12), transparent (13), liquid (14), reddish (15), red-brown (16), | (17), | (18), | (19), | (20)

Cervix — Position and opening

Cervix — Firmness

Intercourse: X (day 4), X (day 6), X (day 17), X (day 19), X (day 21), X (day 24)

Fertile Days

Arbeitsgruppe NFP ©

Identifying the infertile time after ovulation

» **Angelica B. is a pediatric nurse. She has two children and is undecided whether or not she wants to conceive.**

1. Identify the shift in the cervical mucus sign.

2. Are there any disturbances or special circumstances?

3. Identify the earliest first higher temperature reading and enter this in the column on the right.

4. Determine the beginning of the infertile time after ovulation and mark all fertile days with an "F."

| Occurrences Unusual/special disturbances | | | | | | headache | | | | late meal | | | | | | | | | | | | | | | | | | | | | | | | | | | | | | | |

Time: 6³⁰ — 7

| | | | | | | | | | | | | | | | | | | P | 1 | 2 | 3 | | | | | | | | | | | | | | | | | | | | |

Midcycle pain / Breast symptoms

Mucus abbreviation — temperature row markers: + + + + + + (cycle days 11–16), S S S S S S S S S S S (days 6–16), Ø Ø Ø Ø (days 17–20), P at day 17

Basal body temperature scale: 37,5 / 37,4 / 37,3 / 37,2 / 37,1 / 37,0 / 36,9 / 36,8 / 36,7 / 36,6 / 36,5 / 36,4 / 36,3 / 36,2 / 36,1 / 36,0

Count-up numbers near 36,4 line: 6 5 4 3 2 1 (cycle days 8–13)

Cycle day	1	2	3	4	5	6	7	8	9	10	11	12	13	14	15	16	17	18	19	20	21	22	23	24	25	26	27	28	29	30	31	32	33	34	35	36	37	38	39	40
Date: February	4	5	6	7	8	9	10	11	12	13	14	15	16	17	18	19	20	21	22	23	24	25	26	27	28	29	³/₁	2	3	4	5	6	7	8	9	10	11	12	13	14

Menstruation: marks on days 1–6 and around days 18–19, and around day 30

Mucus

Sensation: moist (9), moist (10), moist (11), moist (12), moist (13), wet (14), wet (15), slippery (16), wet (17), wet (18), moist (19), nothing (20), nothing (21), nothing (22)

Appearance: lumpy (9), lumpy (10), sticky (11), thick (12), sticky (13), elastic (14), transparent (15), transparent (16), liquid (17), reddish (18), red-brown (19)

Cervix

Position and opening

Firmness

| Intercourse | | | | X | | X | | | | | | | | | | | X | | X | | X | | | | | X | | | | | | | | | | | | | | |

Fertile Days: → F /

Arbeitsgruppe NFP ©

®

Cycle-no* [ ] [7]

Temperature taken

R [X]
V [ ]
O [ ]

Earliest first higher temperature reading in the previous cycles

[1] [4]

Minus 8 [ ] [ ]

Earliest first higher temperature reading in this cycle

[1] [5]

Do you intend to become pregnant in the next cycle?

yes [ ]
no [ ]
undecided [X]

✳ Malteser
...weil Nähe zählt.

Identifying the infertile time after ovulation

1. The shift of the cervical mucus sign is on cycle day 16.

2. On cycle days 6 and 10, potential disturbances are entered. Since the temperature measurements were not affected, they are not bracketed.

3. The earliest first higher temperature reading is on cycle day 15.

4. The infertile time after ovulation begins on the evening of cycle day 19.

On cycle days 15 and 16 there is light mid-cycle bleeding.

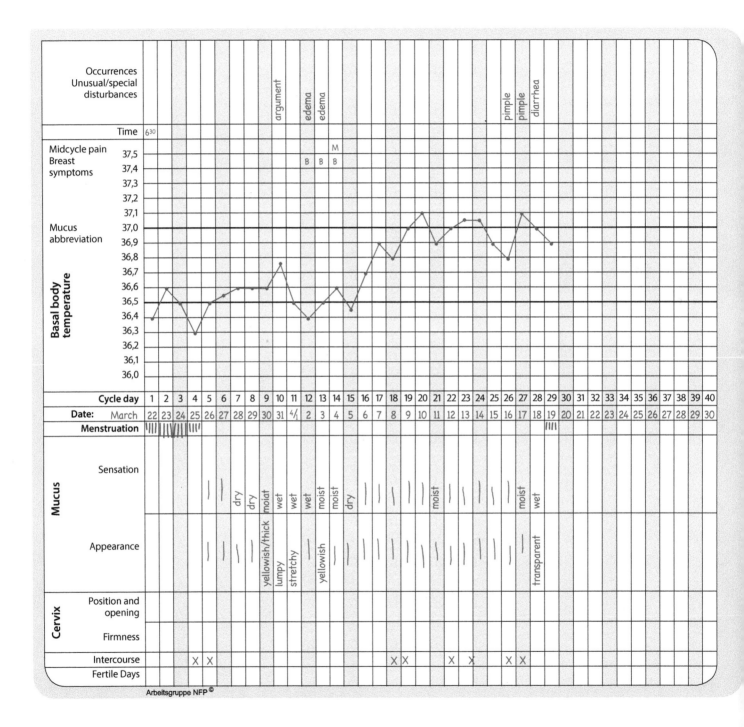

Arbeitsgruppe NFP ©

SENSIPLAN ®

Cycle-no* | 3 | 4

Temperature taken
R | X
V |
O |

Earliest first higher temperature reading in the previous cycles | 1 | 4

Minus 8

Earliest first higher temperature reading in this cycle

Do you intend to become pregnant in the next cycle?

yes |
no | X
undecided |

✠ **Malteser**
...weil Nähe zählt.

Identifying the infertile time after ovulation

» Kirsten O. is a 27-year-old medical assistant with no children. She is not trying to conceive and has been using Sensiplan for about three years.

1. Enter the cervical mucus abbreviations and identify the shift in the cervical mucus sign.

2. Are there any disturbances or special circumstances?

3. Identify the earliest first higher temperature reading and enter this in the column on the right.

4. Identify the beginning of the infertile time after ovulation.

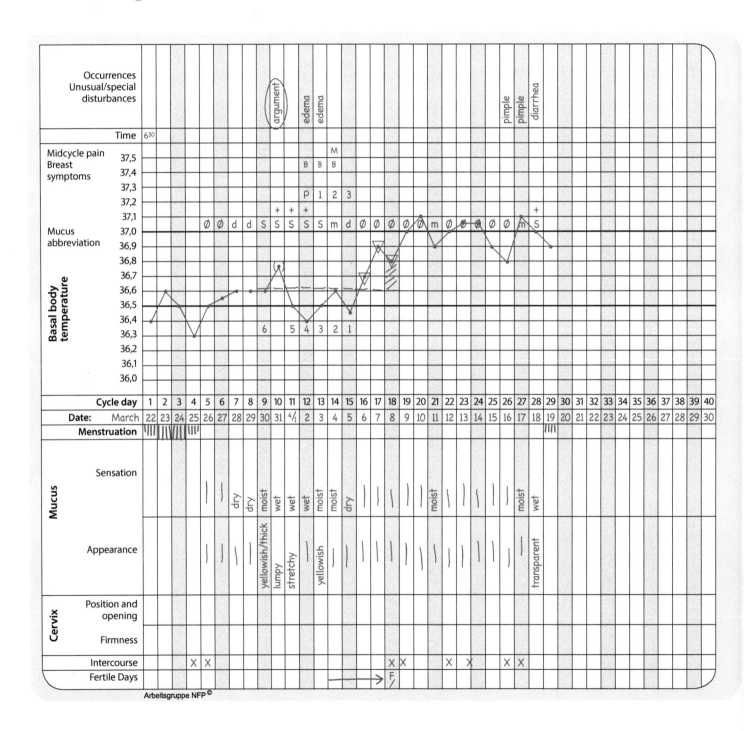

Arbeitsgruppe NFP ©

Identifying the infertile time after ovulation

1. The shift of the cervical mucus sign is on cycle day 12.

2. On cycle day 10 an argument is entered as a disturbance, which leads to a rise in temperature. The value is put in brackets and does not count when counting back over the previous six lower measurements. Kirsten O. notes water retention (edema) as a disturbance on cycle days 12 and 13 of the cycle, however, her temperature measurements on these days were not affected and measurements are not bracketed.

3. The earliest first higher temperature reading is on cycle day 16.

4. The infertile time after ovulation begins on the evening of cycle day 18.

®

Cycle-no* | 3 | 4

Temperature taken
R X
V
O

Earliest first higher temperature reading in the previous cycles
| 1 | 4 |

Minus 8 | | |

Earliest first higher temperature reading in this cycle | 1 | 6 |

Do you intend to become pregnant in the next cycle?
yes
no X
undecided

Malteser
...weil Nähe zählt.

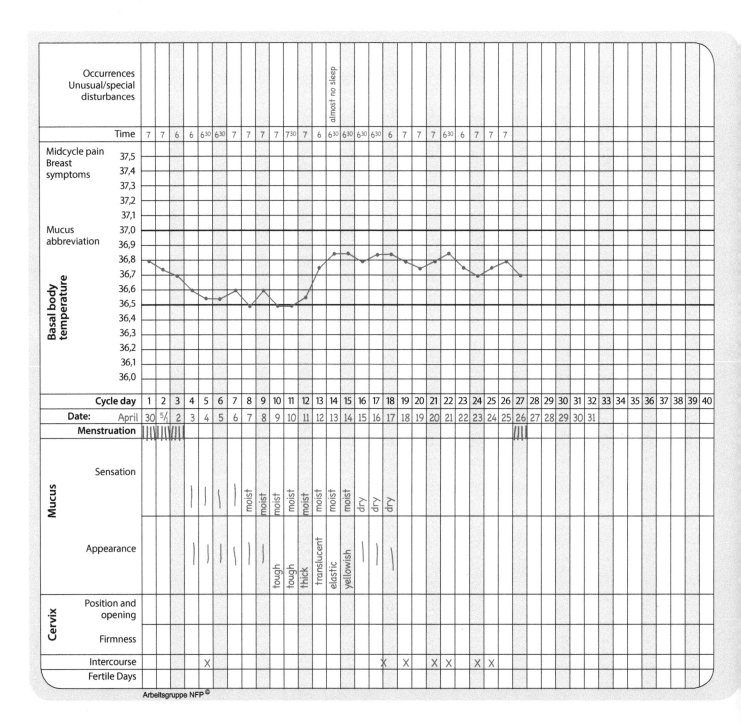

Arbeitsgruppe NFP ©

sensiplan ®

Cycle-no* | 1 | 7 |

Temperature taken

R

V X

O

Earliest first higher
temperature reading
in the previous cycles

| 1 | 3 |

Minus 8

Earliest first higher
temperature
reading in
this cycle

Do you intend to
become pregnant
in the next cycle?

yes

no X

undecided

✳ **Malteser**
...weil Nähe zählt.

Identifying the infertile time after ovulation

» **Sabine B. is a 32-year-old teacher. She has no children and would like to have children in about one year.**

1. Enter the cervical mucus abbreviations and identify the shift in the cervical mucus sign.

2. Are there any disturbances or special circumstances?

3. Identify the earliest first higher temperature reading and enter this in the column on the right.

4. Identify the beginning of the infertile time after ovulation.

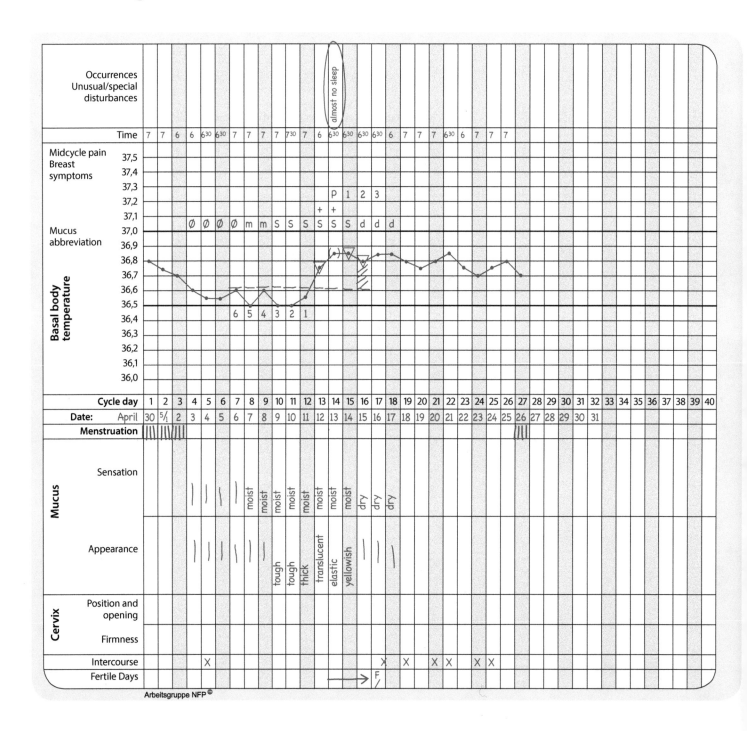

Arbeitsgruppe NFP ©

®

Cycle-no* | 1 | 7

Temperature taken
R
V | X
O

Earliest first higher temperature reading in the previous cycles

1 | 3

Minus 8

Earliest first higher temperature reading in this cycle

1 | 3

Do you intend to become pregnant in the next cycle?

yes
no | X
undecided

✳ **Malteser**
...weil Nähe zählt.

Identifying the infertile time after ovulation

1. The shift of the cervical mucus sign is on cycle day 14.

2. On cycle day 14 the disturbance "almost no sleep" is entered. It is not clear if this temperature measurement is increased because of the lack of sleep or if it represents a true higher measurement. Therefore, the measurement is put in brackets.

3. The earliest first higher temperature reading is on cycle day 13 in this cycle.

4. The infertile time after ovulation begins on the evening of cycle day 17.

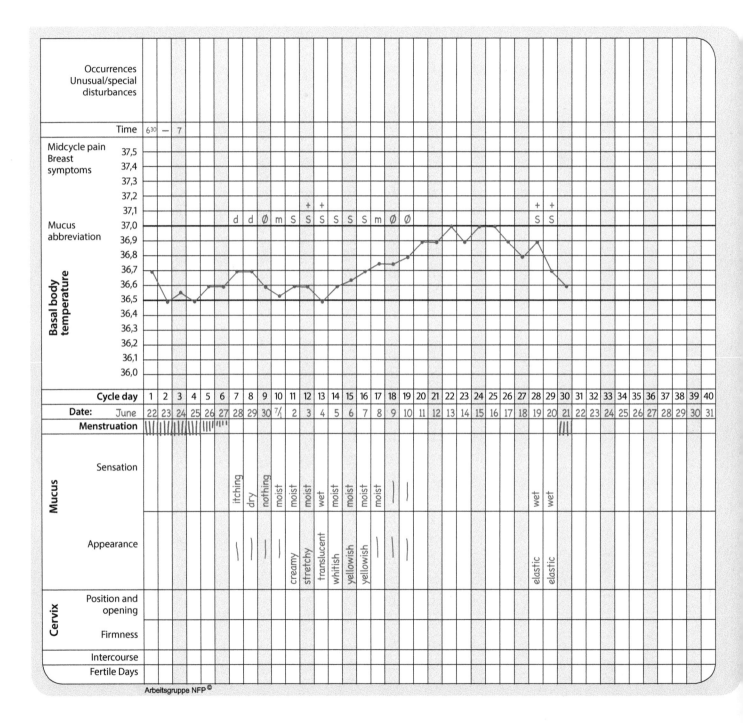

Arbeitsgruppe NFP ©

sensiplan ®

Cycle-no*		1	8

Temperature taken	R	X
	V	
	O	

Earliest first higher temperature reading in the previous cycles

	1	6

Minus 8

Earliest first higher temperature reading in this cycle

Do you intend to become pregnant in the next cycle?

yes	
no	X
undecided	

✳ Malteser
...weil Nähe zählt.

Identifying the infertile time after ovulation

» **Daniela W. is a 26-year-old cosmetologist.**

1. Identify the shift in the cervical mucus sign.

2. Are there any disturbances or special circumstances?

3. Identify the earliest first higher temperature reading and enter this in the column on the right.

4. Identify the beginning of the infertile time after ovulation.

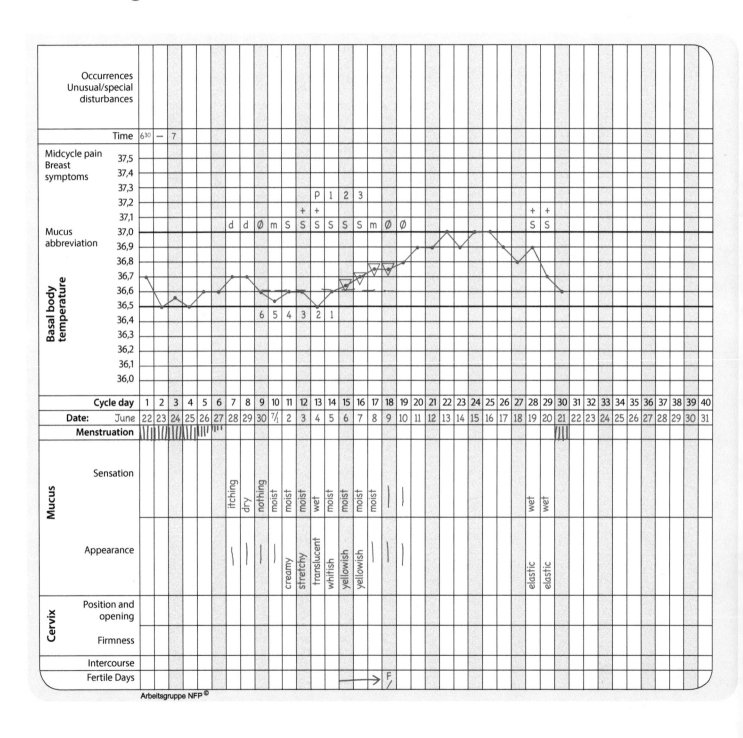

Arbeitsgruppe NFP ©

®

Cycle-no* | 1 | 8

Temperature taken

R | X
V |
O |

Earliest first higher temperature reading in the previous cycles

1 | 6

Minus 8

Earliest first higher temperature reading in this cycle | 1 | 5

Do you intend to become pregnant in the next cycle?

yes |
no | X
undecided |

✴ **Malteser**
...weil Nähe zählt.

Identifying the infertile time after ovulation

1. The shift of the cervical mucus sign is on cycle day 13.

2. No disturbances or special circumstances are recorded.

3. The earliest first higher temperature reading is on cycle day 15, one day earlier than any previous earliest first higher temperature reading.

4. The infertile time after ovulation begins on the evening of cycle day 18.

Note:
- The temperature is evaluated using the first exception to the rule.

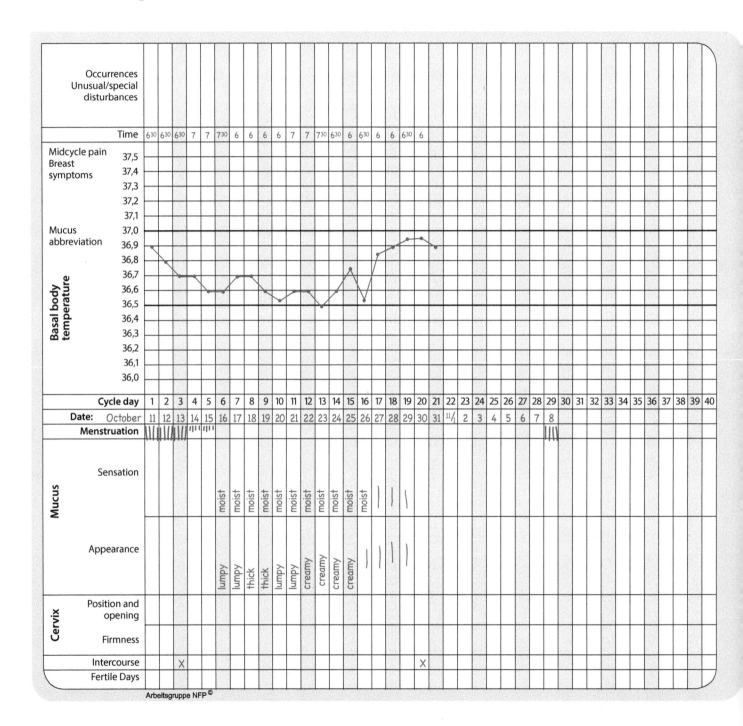

		1	2	3	4	5	6	7	8	9	10	11	12	13	14	15	16	17	18	19	20	21	22

Occurrences Unusual/special disturbances

| Time | 6³⁰ | 6³⁰ | 6³⁰ | 7 | 7 | 7³⁰ | 6 | 6 | 6 | 6 | 7 | 7 | 7³⁰ | 6³⁰ | 6 | 6³⁰ | 6 | 6 | 6³⁰ | 6 |

Midcycle pain / Breast symptoms

Mucus abbreviation

Basal body temperature (°C): 37,5 – 36,0

Cycle day	1	2	3	4	5	6	7	8	9	10	11	12	13	14	15	16	17	18	19	20	21	22	23	24	25	26	27	28	29	30	31	32	33	34	35	36	37	38	39	40

Date: October 11 12 13 14 15 16 17 18 19 20 21 22 23 24 25 26 27 28 29 30 31 ¹¹/₁ 2 3 4 5 6 7 8

Menstruation

Mucus

Sensation: moist (days 6–17)

Appearance: lumpy, lumpy, thick, thick, lumpy, lumpy, creamy, creamy, creamy, creamy (days 6–15)

Cervix

Position and opening

Firmness

Intercourse: X (day 3), X (day 19)

Fertile Days

Arbeitsgruppe NFP ©

Cycle-no* | 2

Temperature taken R X
V
O

Earliest first higher
temperature reading
in the previous cycles

| 1 | 7 |

Minus 8

Earliest first higher
temperature
reading in
this cycle

Do you intend to
become pregnant
in the next cycle?

yes
no X
undecided

Malteser
...weil Nähe zählt.

Identifying the infertile time after ovulation

» **Stephanie W. is a 22-year-old administrator. She has no children and would like to avoid getting pregnant.**

1. Enter the cervical mucus abbreviations and identify the shift in the cervical mucus sign.

2. Are there any disturbances or special circumstances?

3. Identify the earliest first higher temperature reading and enter this in the column on the right.

4. Identify the beginning of the infertile time after ovulation.

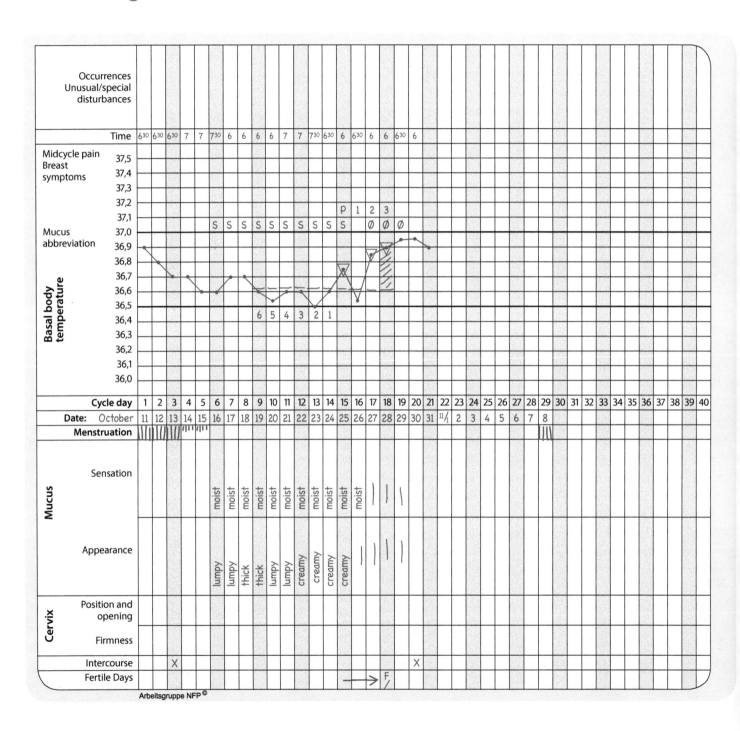

Arbeitsgruppe NFP ©

Cycle-no* | | | 2 |

Temperature taken

R [X]
V [ ]
O [ ]

Earliest first higher
temperature reading
in the previous cycles

| 1 | 7 |

Minus 8 | | |

Earliest first higher
temperature
reading in | 1 | 5 |
this cycle

Do you intend to
become pregnant
in the next cycle?

yes [ ]
no [X]
undecided [ ]

Identifying the infertile time after ovulation

1. The shift of the cervical mucus sign is on cycle day 15.

2. No disturbances or special circumstances are recorded.

3. The earliest first higher temperature reading is on cycle day 15, two days earlier than any previous earliest first higher temperature reading.

4. The infertile time after ovulation begins on the evening of cycle day 18.

Notes:
- The temperature is evaluated using the second exception to the rule.
- In this cycle, no S+ quality cervical mucus is observed. However, a shift can still be identified.

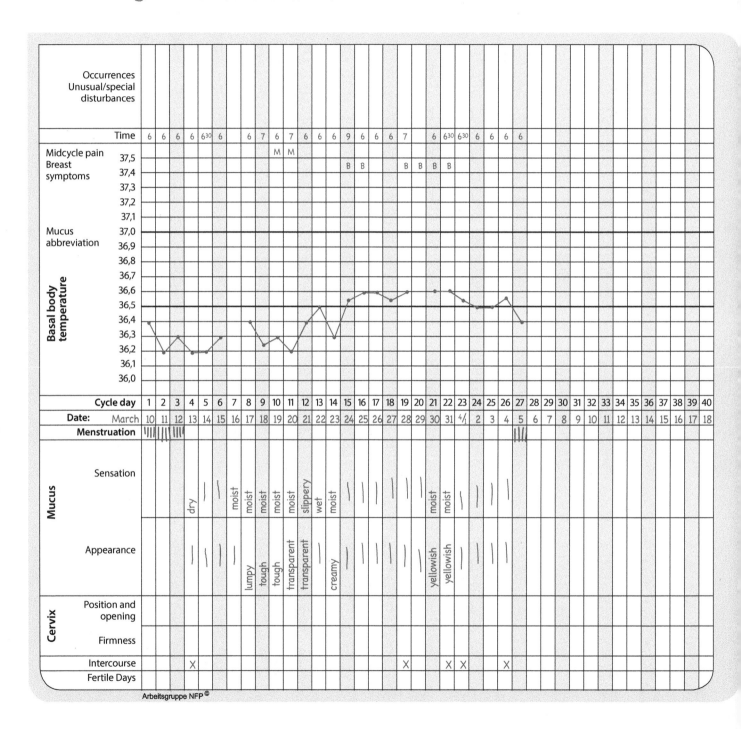

Cycle day	1	2	3	4	5	6	7	8	9	10	11	12	13	14	15	16	17	18	19	20	21	22	23	24	25	26	27	28	29	30	31	32	33	34	35	36	37	38	39	40
Date: March	10	11	12	13	14	15	16	17	18	19	20	21	22	23	24	25	26	27	28	29	30	31	4/1	2	3	4	5	6	7	8	9	10	11	12	13	14	15	16	17	18

Arbeitsgruppe NFP ©

SENSIPLAN ®

Cycle-no* | | 7 |

Temperature taken
R | |
V | X |
O | |

Earliest first higher temperature reading in the previous cycles

| 1 | 3 |

Minus 8 | |

Earliest first higher temperature reading in this cycle | |

Do you intend to become pregnant in the next cycle?

yes | |
no | X |
undecided | |

✳ **Malteser**
...weil Nähe zählt.

Identifying the infertile time after ovulation

» Olivia E. is a 29-year-old part-time employee. She has one child.

1. Enter the cervical mucus abbreviations and identify the shift in the cervical mucus sign.

2. Are there any disturbances or special circumstances?

3. Identify the earliest first higher temperature reading and enter this in the column on the right.

4. Identify the beginning of the infertile time after ovulation.

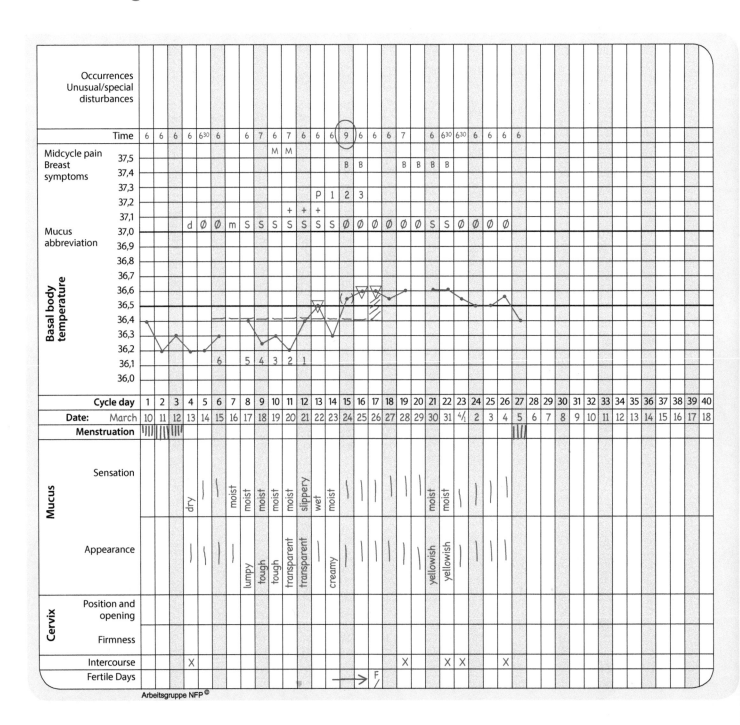

Arbeitsgruppe NFP ©

Identifying the infertile time after ovulation

1. The shift of the cervical mucus sign is on cycle day 13.

2. The temperature measurement on cycle day 15 is a disturbance and is put in brackets. The disturbance is noted because the temperature was taken later than usual.

3. The missing value on cycle day 7 is not taken into account when counting the six previous lower temperatures.

4. The earliest first higher temperature reading is on cycle day 13.

5. The infertile time after ovulation begins on the evening of cycle day 17.

Notes:
- The temperature is evaluated using the second exception to the rule.
- If Olivia E. noticed in the previous cycles that measuring later does not affect the temperature, she does not have to put the temperature reading on cycle day 15 in brackets.

®

Cycle-no* | 7

Temperature taken
R
V | X
O

Earliest first higher temperature reading in the previous cycles | 1 3

Minus 8

Earliest first higher temperature reading in this cycle | 1 3

Do you intend to become pregnant in the next cycle?

yes
no | X
undecided

✠ **Malteser**
...weil Nähe zählt.

Training 14   The infertile time after ovulation

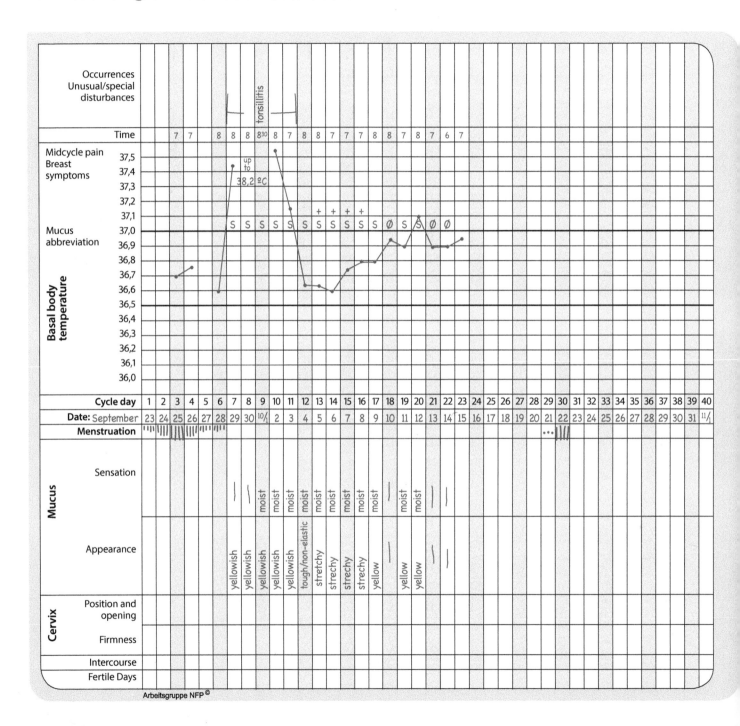

Identifying the infertile time after ovulation

» **Eliza S. is a 24-year-old business administration student.**

1. Identify the shift in the cervical mucus sign.

2. Are there any disturbances or special circumstances?

3. Identify the earliest first higher temperature reading and enter this in the column on the right.

4. Identify the beginning of the infertile time after ovulation.

---

sensiplan ®

Cycle-no*   1 5

Temperature taken   R X
                     V
                     O

Earliest first higher temperature reading in the previous cycles   1 6

Minus 8

Earliest first higher temperature reading in this cycle

Do you intend to become pregnant in the next cycle?

yes
no X
undecided

✳ **Malteser**
...weil Nähe zählt.

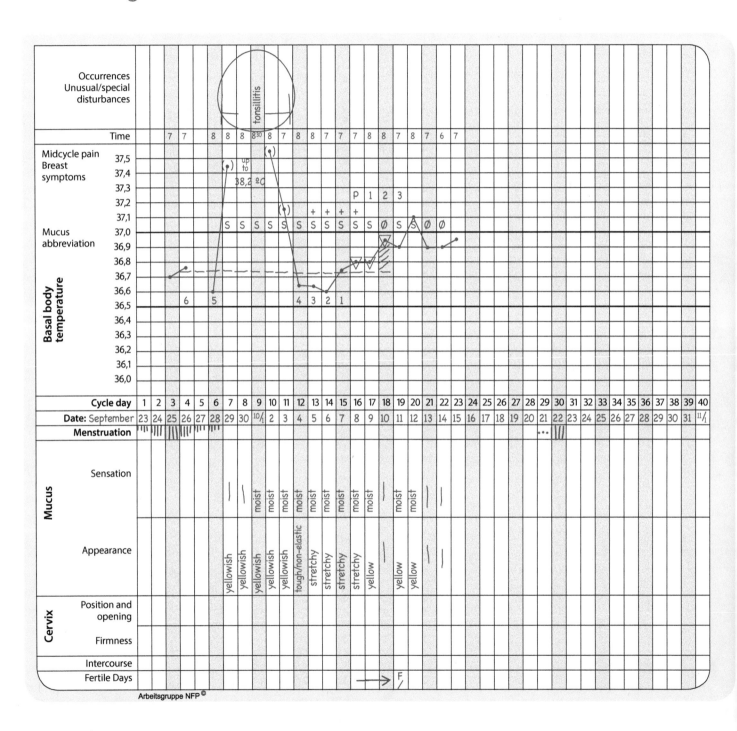

Identifying the infertile time after ovulation

1. The shift of the cervical mucus sign is on cycle day 16.

2. On cycle days 7-11 Eliza has tonsillitis and a fever. These temperatures are put in brackets and not taken into account when counting the six previous lower temperatures.

3. The earliest first higher temperature reading is on cycle day 16.

4. The infertile time after ovulation begins on the evening of cycle day 19.

®

Cycle-no*   ☐ 1 5

Temperature taken
R ☒
V ☐
O ☐

Earliest first higher temperature reading in the previous cycles
1 6

Minus 8   ☐☐

Earliest first higher temperature reading in this cycle
1 6

Do you intend to become pregnant in the next cycle?

yes ☐
no ☒
undecided ☐

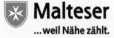

Malteser
...weil Nähe zählt.

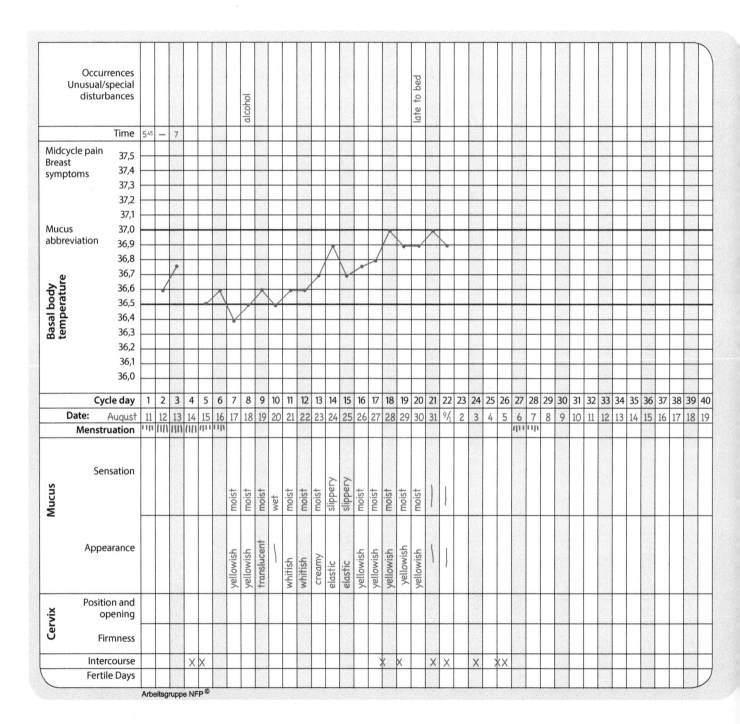

Occurrences Unusual/special disturbances			alcohol ... late to bed

Time	5⁴⁵ — 7

Basal body temperature (°C): Midcycle pain / Breast symptoms / Mucus abbreviation
Scale: 37,5 / 37,4 / 37,3 / 37,2 / 37,1 / 37,0 / 36,9 / 36,8 / 36,7 / 36,6 / 36,5 / 36,4 / 36,3 / 36,2 / 36,1 / 36,0

Cycle day	1	2	3	4	5	6	7	8	9	10	11	12	13	14	15	16	17	18	19	20	21	22	23	24	25	26	27	28	29	30	31	32	33	34	35	36	37	38	39	40
Date: August	11	12	13	14	15	16	17	18	19	20	21	22	23	24	25	26	27	28	29	30	31	9/1	2	3	4	5	6	7	8	9	10	11	12	13	14	15	16	17	18	19
Menstruation	‖	‖	‖	‖	‖	‖																					‖	‖												

Mucus

Sensation: (cd 7) moist, (8) moist, (9) moist, (10) wet, (11) moist, (12) moist, (13) moist, (14) slippery, (15) slippery, (16) moist, (17) moist, (18) moist, (19) moist, (20) moist

Appearance: (cd 7) yellowish, (8) yellowish, (9) translucent, (10) \ , (11) whitish, (12) whitish, (13) creamy, (14) elastic, (15) elastic, (16) yellowish, (17) yellowish, (18) yellowish, (19) yellowish, (20) yellowish

Cervix
Position and opening
Firmness

| Intercourse | | | | X | X | | | | | | | | | | | | | X | X | | X | X | | X | X | X | | | | | |

Fertile Days

Arbeitsgruppe NFP ©

SENSIPLAN ®

Cycle-no* | 1 | 9

Temperature taken
R | X
V |
O |

Earliest first higher temperature reading in the previous cycles

1 | 3

Minus 8 | |

Earliest first higher temperature reading in this cycle | |

Do you intend to become pregnant in the next cycle?

yes |
no | X
undecided |

✵ Malteser
...weil Nähe zählt.

Identifying the infertile time after ovulation

» Corinna L. is a 31-year-old salesperson. She has two children, and would like to avoid getting pregnant.

1. Enter the cervical mucus abbreviations and identify the shift in the cervical mucus sign.

2. Are there any disturbances or special circumstances?

3. Identify the earliest first higher temperature reading and enter this in the column on the right.

4. Identify the beginning of the infertile time after ovulation.

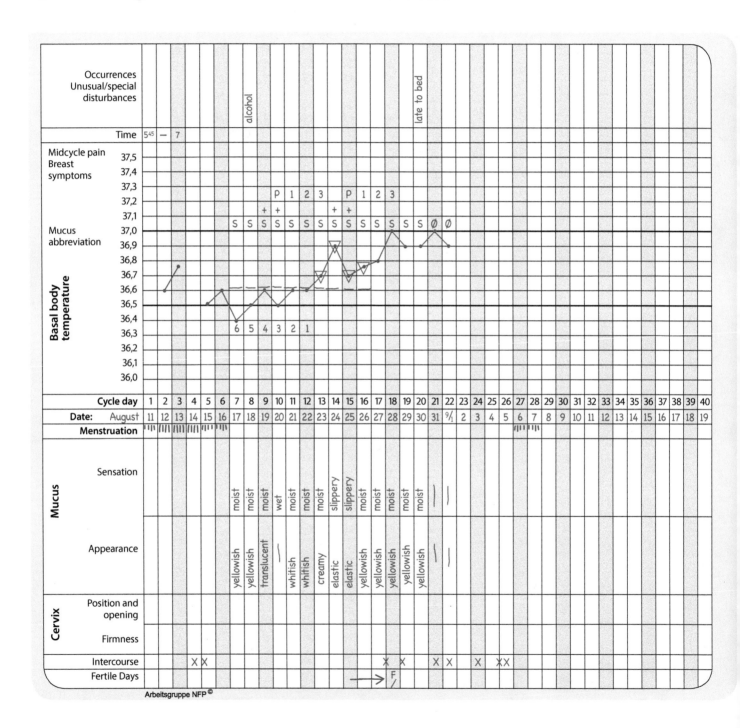

Identifying the infertile time after ovulation

1. There are two shifts in the cervical mucus sign - on cycle days 10 and 15.

2. Alcohol on cycle day 8 does not affect the temperature and is not bracketed.

3. Cycle day 20 shows "late to bed," however, it is not considered a disturbance because the evaluation had already been done.

4. The earliest first higher temperature reading is on cycle day 13.

5. The infertile time after ovulation begins on the evening of cycle day 18.

Notes:
- The temperature is evaluated using the first exception to the rule.
- The mucus shift on cycle day 15 is used for the double check because the best quality cervical mucus is present again before the temperature evaluation has been completed.

®

Cycle-no*   1   9

Temperature taken   R [X]
   V [ ]
   O [ ]

Earliest first higher temperature reading in the previous cycles
   1   3

Minus 8   [   ]

Earliest first higher temperature reading in this cycle
   1   3

Do you intend to become pregnant in the next cycle?

yes [ ]
no [X]
undecided [ ]

✠ **Malteser**
...weil Nähe zählt.

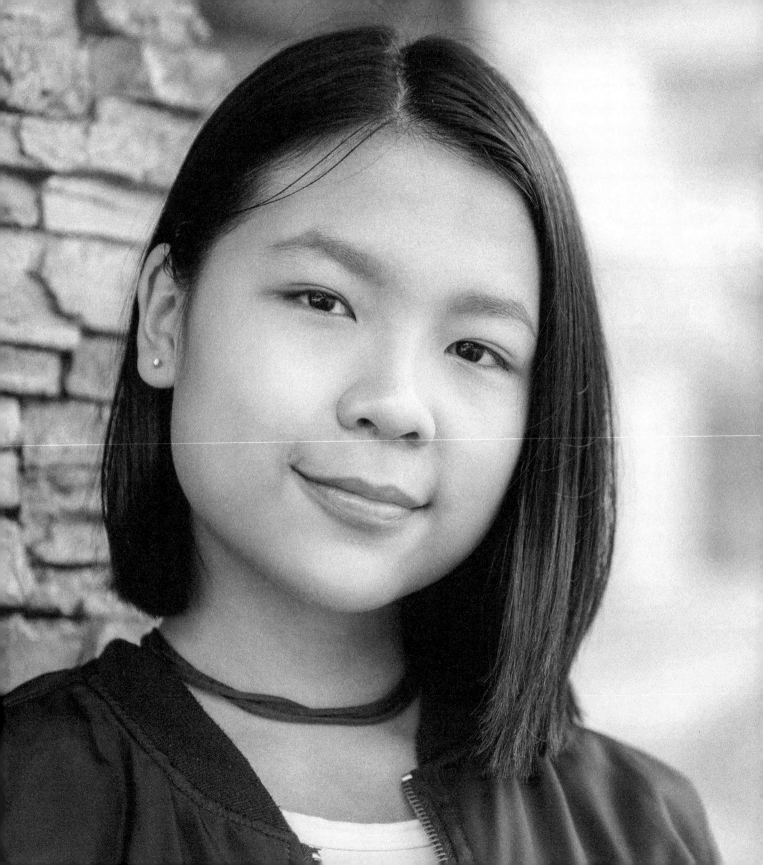

Chapter 3

The infertile time at the beginning of the cycle

The infertile time at the beginning of the cycle (before ovulation) is identified using cervical mucus and either the Minus-8 Rule or the 5-Day Rule, whichever is first. The length of the pre-ovulatory time is often determined by using information obtained from previous cycles. This chapter explains the Minus-8 and 5-Day Rules in more detail and how to apply them using several practice charts.

Identifying the infertile time at the beginning of the cycle

The infertile time before ovulation is more challenging to identify than the infertile time after ovulation and may only be assumed if there has been a temperature shift in the previous cycle (cf. manual *Natural & Safe: The Handbook*). Because a new Sensiplan user may have limited information about her previous cycles, in the first cycle using Sensiplan, the user must assume she is fertile starting on cycle day 1. In subsequent cycles, the beginning of the fertile time before ovulation is determined using cervical mucus in double check with either the Minus-8 Rule or the 5-Day Rule, whichever is first (cf. manual *Natural & Safe: The Handbook*).

5-Day Rule:

The first 5 cycle days can be assumed to be infertile days unless cervical mucus is noted or the Minus-8 Rule begins fertility first.

During your previous 12 cycles, if the earliest first higher temperature reading has ever been on or before cycle day 12, "the first 5 days of infertility" no longer applies. From that point on, the "earliest first higher temperature reading Minus-8 Rule will apply.

The Minus-8 Rule:

The last infertile day at the beginning of the cycle is the day of the earliest first higher temperature reading from at least 12 previous cycle charts Minus-8 days. If you observe cervical mucus or feel "moist" before this day, the fertile phase starts immediately using the double check principle of "whichever is first" (cf. manual *Natural & Safe: The Handbook*).

Sensiplan for the beginner:

• In the first learning cycle, fertility is assumed starting on cycle day 1.

• In each cycle following a temperature shift, the earliest first higher temperature reading for that cycle is entered in the column on the right.

• If a temperature shift can be evaluated, the 5-day rule may be applied in the next cycle, i.e., the first 5 days are considered infertile.

• Mark the first 5 infertile days at the beginning of the cycle by drawing a box around cycle day 5 and a vertical line between cycle days 5 and 6

• If cervical mucus signs occur earlier, the fertile phase begins immediately, using the double check principle of "whichever is first."

• The earliest first higher temperature reading from all previous cycles is also entered in the right-hand column at the beginning of each new cycle.

• With each cycle, pay attention to whether the earliest first higher temperature reading is earlier than in previous cycles. If so, this must be entered as the earliest first higher temperature in all future cycles.

• If the earliest first higher temperature was once on cycle day 12 or earlier over the past 12 cycles, "the first 5 days" rule no longer applies. In future cycles, you will need to use "the earliest first higher temperature reading Minus-8" Rule (cf. manual *Natural & Safe: The Handbook*).

Once the Sensiplan user completes 12 cycles of temperature shift evaluations, she proceeds as follows:

• At the beginning of the 13th cycle, the earliest first higher temperature reading from all previous cycles is entered in the column on the right.

• Subtract 8 days. This gives you the number of infertile days at the beginning of the cycle (example: 15-8 = 7).

• Draw a box around the number and a vertical line to the right of the box that extends to the bottom of the cycle chart. Days to the left of the line are considered infertile; days to the right of the line are considered fertile.

• The first fertile day is recorded with an "F" on the row marked "Fertile days." All other fertile days are then marked with an "F" until the end of the fertile time can be identified.

• If the cervical mucus sign is present before the verticle line, the fertile time begins immediately, using the double check principle of "whichever is first."

• After the temperature evaluation is complete, the earliest first higher temperature reading in this cycle is entered in the column on the right side of the chart and compared to previous first higher temperature readings.

Another option for a double check is to identify the infertile time at the beginning of the cycle by observing temperature and the cervix.

Rule: Cervix

As long as the cervix is unchanged after menstruation, you can assume that you are infertile, providing the 5-Day Rule or the Minus-8 Rule has not already signaled fertility. If there is a change of the feeling or position of the cervix at the beginning of the cycle, the fertile phase begins immediately.

Special rules for the menstruation calendar:

If you have kept a menstruation diary before using Sensiplan, you may have the option of prolonging the infertile time at the beginning of the cycle, using the Minus-20-Rule.

The Minus-20 Rule:

To use the Minus-20 Rule, find your shortest cycle length from at least 12 previously recorded cycles and subtract 20 days to identify your last infertile day at the beginning of the cycle. If you observe cervical mucus before this day, the fertile phase starts immediately using the double check principle of "whichever is first."

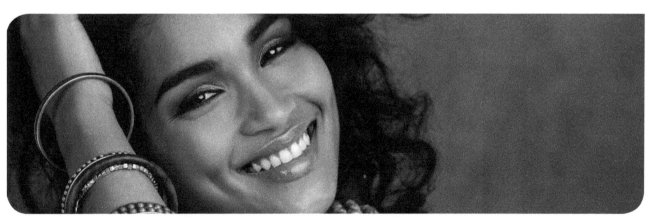

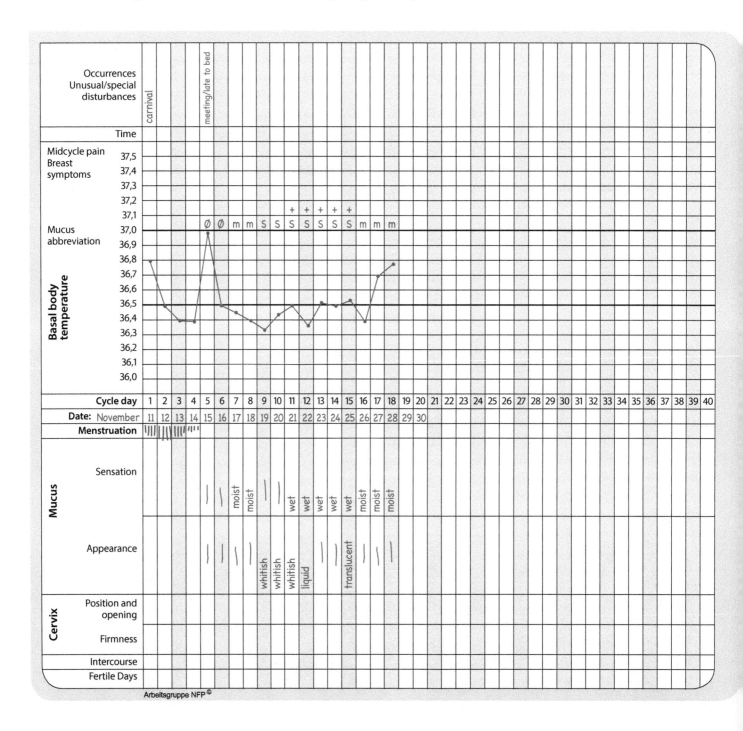

Arbeitsgruppe NFP ©

Identifying the infertile time at the beginning of the cycle

» Karen J. is a 38-year-old mother of two children. This is her first cycle using Sensiplan.

1. Identify the last infertile day at the beginning of the cycle and mark the first fertile day with "F."

2. Are there any disturbances or special circumstances?

Cycle-no* 1

Temperature taken R
V X
O

Earliest first higher temperature reading in the previous cycles

Minus 8

Earliest first higher temperature reading in this cycle

Do you intend to become pregnant in the next cycle?

yes
no X
undecided

✳ **Malteser**
...weil Nähe zählt.

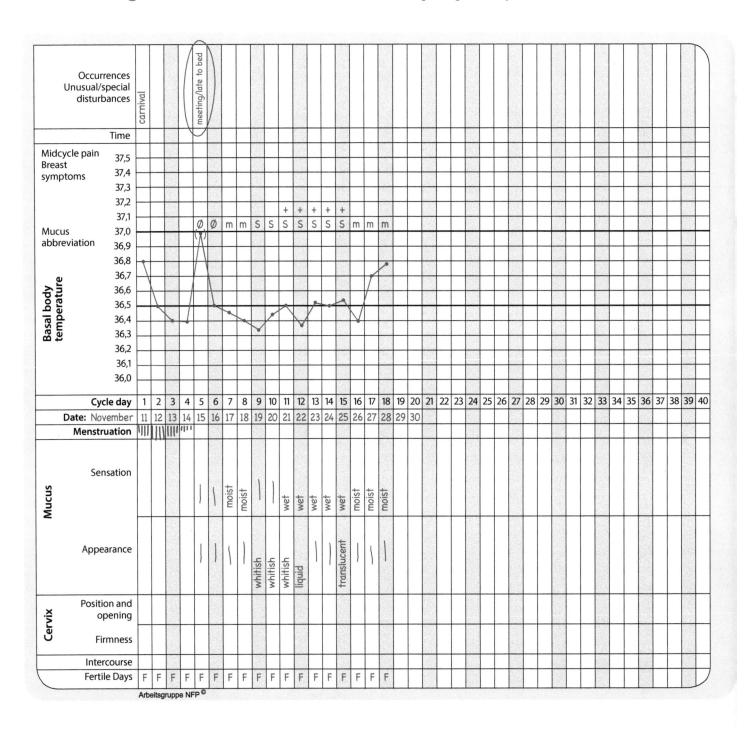

Arbeitsgruppe NFP ©

®

Cycle-no* | | 1 |

Temperature taken

R | |
V | X |
O | |

Earliest first higher
temperature reading
in the previous cycles

| / |

Minus 8 | | |

Earliest first higher
temperature
reading in
this cycle | | |

Do you intend to
become pregnant
in the next cycle?

yes | |
no | X |
undecided | |

✳ **Malteser**
...weil Nähe zählt.

Identifying the infertile time at the beginning of the cycle

1. Because Karen J. is in her first cycle using Sensiplan and has no prior charting experience, she must assume that she is fertile starting on cycle day 1 of this cycle.

2. The temperature measurement on cycle day 5 is a disturbance ("meeting/late to bed") and is put in brackets.

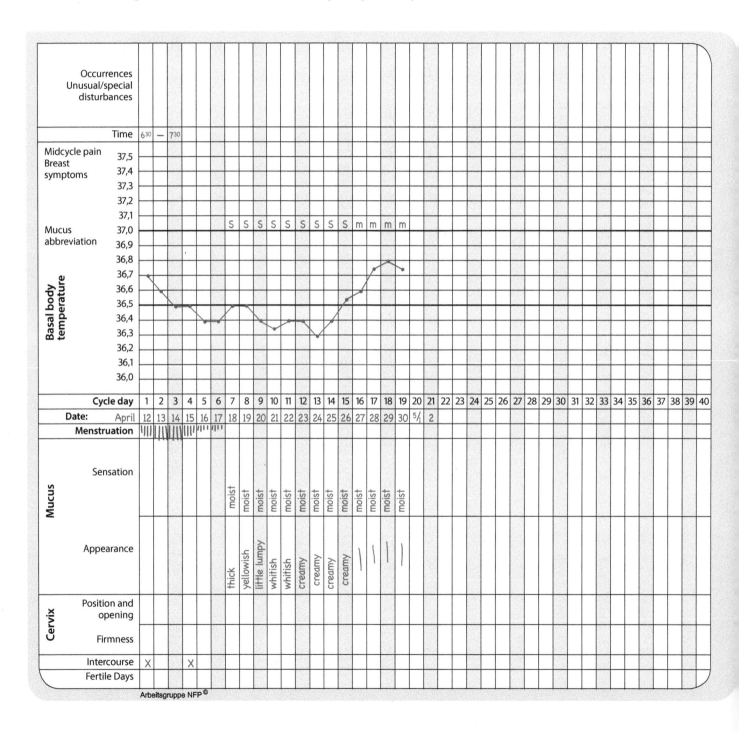

	Cycle day	1	2	3	4	5	6	7	8	9	10	11	12	13	14	15	16	17	18	19	20	21	22	23	24	25	26	27	28	29	30	31	32	33	34	35	36	37	38	39	40
Date:	April	12	13	14	15	16	17	18	19	20	21	22	23	24	25	26	27	28	29	30	5/1	2																			

Mucus abbreviation: S S S S S S S S S m m m m

Menstruation (days 1–6)

Mucus Sensation: moist (days 7–19)

Mucus Appearance: thick, yellowish, little lumpy, whitish, whitish, creamy, creamy, creamy, creamy, \ \ | \

Intercourse: X (day 1), X (day 4)

Arbeitsgruppe NFP ©

Identifying the infertile time at the beginning of the cycle

» Julia K. is a 26-year-old administrator and has one child. This is her seventh cycle using Sensiplan. She observed a temperature shift in her sixth cycle.

1. Identify the last infertile day at the beginning of the cycle and mark the first fertile day with "F."

2. Identify the shift in the cervical mucus sign.

3. Are there any disturbances or special circumstances?

4. Identify the earliest first higher temperature reading and enter this in the column on the right.

5. Identify the beginning of the infertile time after ovulation.

6. Record the earliest first higher temperature reading.

---

sensiplan ®

Cycle-no* [ ] 7

Temperature taken
R [ ]
V [ ]
O X

Earliest first higher temperature reading in the previous cycles
1 6

Minus 8 [ ]

Earliest first higher temperature reading in this cycle [ ]

Do you intend to become pregnant in the next cycle?

yes [ ]
no X
undecided [ ]

✳ Malteser
...weil Nähe zählt.

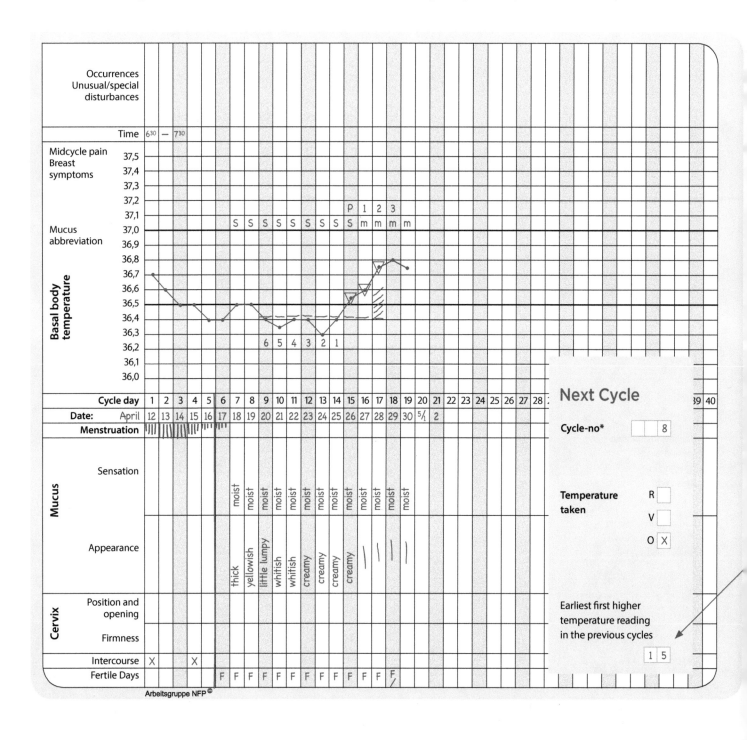

®

Cycle-no* [ ] [7]

Temperature taken

R [ ]

V [ ]

O [X]

Earliest first higher temperature reading in the previous cycles

[1][6]

Minus 8 [⟋]

Earliest first higher temperature reading in this cycle

[1][5]

Do you intend to become pregnant in the next cycle?

yes [ ]

no [X]

undecided [ ]

✳ Malteser
...weil Nähe zählt.

Identifying the infertile time at the beginning of the cycle

1. The infertile phase at the beginning of the cycle was identified using the 5-day rule in double check with the cervical mucus sign. The last infertile day is cycle day 5.

2. The shift of the cervical mucus sign is on cycle day 15.

3. No disturbances or special circumstances are recorded.

4. The earliest first higher temperature reading is on cycle day 15, one day earlier than any previous earliest first higher temperature reading.

5. The infertile time after ovulation begins on the evening of cycle day 18.

6. The earliest first higher temperature reading this cycle has caused a shift from cycle day 16 to cycle day 15 in future cycles.

		1	2	3	4	5	6	7	8	9	10	11	12
Occurrences Unusual/special disturbances						headache							
Time		6⁴⁵	6⁴⁵	6³⁰	7	10	7	6⁴⁵	6³⁰	6	9	6³⁰	6³⁰

Midcycle pain / Breast symptoms

Mucus abbreviation

Basal body temperature (°C): 37,5 · 37,4 · 37,3 · 37,2 · 37,1 · 37,0 · 36,9 · 36,8 · 36,7 · 36,6 · 36,5 · 36,4 · 36,3 · 36,2 · 36,1 · 36,0

Cycle day	1	2	3	4	5	6	7	8	9	10	11	12	13	14	15	16	17	18	19	20	21	22	23	24	25	26	27	28	29	30	31	32	33	34	35	36	37	38	39	40
Date: August	12	13	14	15	16	17	18	19	20	21	22	23	24	25	26	27	28	29	30	31	9/1	2	3	4	5	6	7	8	9	10	11	12	13	14	15	16	17	18	19	20
Menstruation	∥∥∥	∥∥	∥∥∥	∥∥∣	∣∥∣	∥∣∣																																		

Mucus

Sensation						dry	nothing	nothing	moist	moist	moist	wet
Appearance						∣	∣	∣	sticky	translucent	stretchy	

Cervix

Position and opening												
Firmness												
Intercourse						X		X				
Fertile Days												

SENSIPLAN®

Cycle-no* 1 3

Temperature taken R X / V / O

Earliest first higher temperature reading in the previous cycles 1 8

Minus 8

Earliest first higher temperature reading in this cycle

Do you intend to become pregnant in the next cycle?

yes

no X

undecided

Malteser ...weil Nähe zählt.

Identifying the infertile time at the beginning of the cycle

» **Vanessa N. is a 24-year-old journalist. She has been using Sensiplan for more than a year. She observed a temperature shift in her last cycle.**

1. Identify the last infertile day at the beginning of the cycle and mark the first fertile day with "F."
2. Are there any disturbances or special circumstances?

Training 18 – Solution The infertile time at the beginning of the cycle

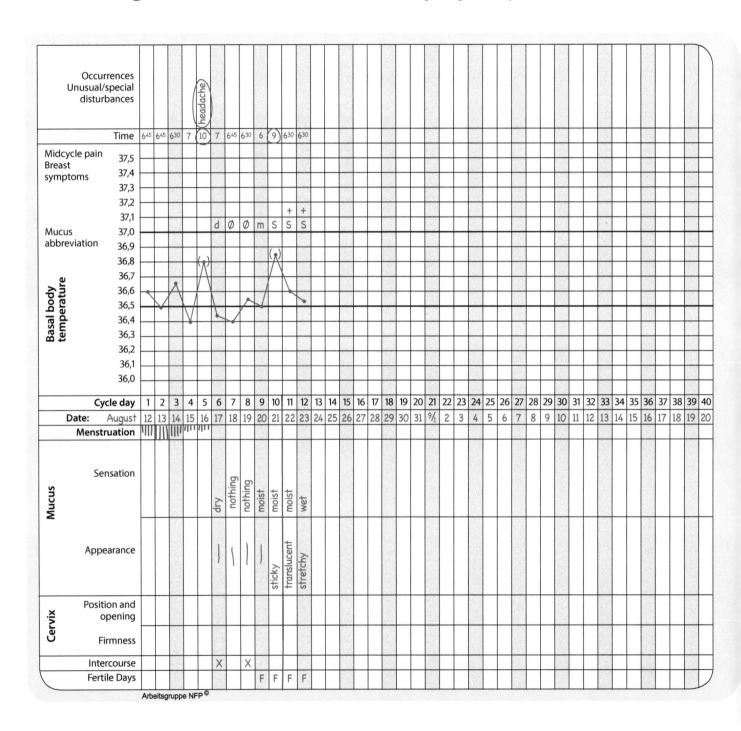

		1	2	3	4	5	6	7	8	9	10	11	12	13	14	15	16	17	18	19	20	21	22	23	24	25	26	27	28	29	30	31	32	33	34	35	36	37	38	39	40

Occurrences Unusual/special disturbances — headache (circled, day 5)

| Time | 6⁴⁵ | 6⁴⁵ | 6³⁰ | 7 | 10 | 7 | 6⁴⁵ | 6³⁰ | 6 | 9 | 6³⁰ | 6³⁰ |

Midcycle pain / Breast symptoms

Mucus abbreviation: d ∅ ∅ m S S S (with + on days 11, 12)

Cycle day: 1–40

Date: August 12 13 14 15 16 17 18 19 20 21 22 23 24 25 26 27 28 29 30 31 9/1 2 3 4 5 6 7 8 9 10 11 12 13 14 15 16 17 18 19 20

Menstruation

Mucus — Sensation: dry, nothing, nothing, moist, moist, moist, wet

Mucus — Appearance: sticky, translucent, stretchy

Cervix — Position and opening

Cervix — Firmness

Intercourse: X (day 6), X (day 8)

Fertile Days: F F F F (days 9–12)

Arbeitsgruppe NFP ©

®

Cycle-no* | 1 | 3

Temperature taken
R | X
V |
O |

Earliest first higher temperature reading in the previous cycles
| 1 | 8

Minus 8 | 1 | 0

Earliest first higher temperature reading in this cycle
| | |

Do you intend to become pregnant in the next cycle?

yes |
no | X
undecided |

Malteser
...weil Nähe zählt.

Identifying the infertile time at the beginning of the cycle

1. Since Vanessa N. has 12 previously recorded temperature shifts, the infertile phase at the beginning of this cycle is identified using the Minus-8 Rule in double check with the cervical mucus sign. The last infertile day at the beginning of the cycle is cycle day 8 because she noticed cervical mucus on cycle days 9 and 10.

2. It appears that for Vanessa N., taking her temperature later than usual affects her temperature measurements on cycle days 5 and 10 and these are counted as disturbances. The headache she reported on cycle day 5 also may have had an effect on her temperature.

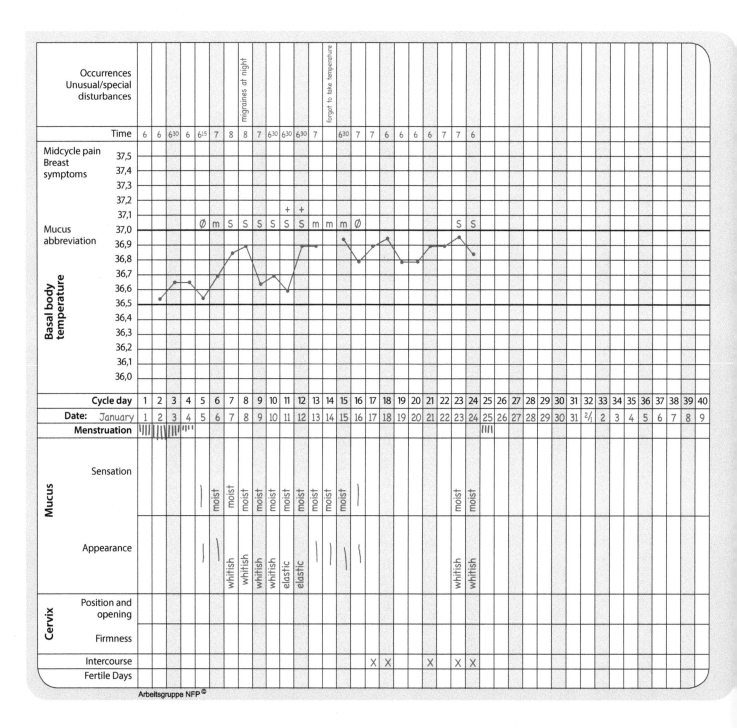

										migraines at night						forgot to take temperature																												

Occurrences Unusual/special disturbances

Time	6	6	6³⁰	6	6¹⁵	7	8	8	7	6³⁰	6³⁰	6³⁰	7		6³⁰	7	7	6	6	6	6	7	7	6																

Midcycle pain
Breast symptoms

Mucus abbreviation: | | | | | Ø | m | S | S | S | S | S | S | m | m | m | Ø | | | | | | S | S |

Temperature markers: + at 37,1 on days 11 and 12

Basal body temperature (°C)

Cycle day	1	2	3	4	5	6	7	8	9	10	11	12	13	14	15	16	17	18	19	20	21	22	23	24	25	26	27	28	29	30	31	32	33	34	35	36	37	38	39	40
Date: January	1	2	3	4	5	6	7	8	9	10	11	12	13	14	15	16	17	18	19	20	21	22	23	24	25	26	27	28	29	30	31	²/₁	2	3	4	5	6	7	8	9
Menstruation	║║║║	║║║║	║║║║	║║║║	║║║║																				║║║║															

Mucus

Sensation:
| | | | |) | moist | moist | moist | moist | moist | moist | moist | moist | moist | moist |) | | | | | | moist | moist | | | | | | | | | | | | | | | | | |

Appearance:
| | | | |) |) | whitish | whitish | whitish | whitish | elastic | elastic |) |) |) |) | | | | | | whitish | whitish | | | | | | | | | | | | | | | | | |

Cervix

Position and opening

Firmness

| Intercourse | | | | | | | | | | | | | | | | X | X | | X | | X | X | | | | | | | | | | | | | | | | | | |
| Fertile Days | | | | | | | | | | | | | | | | | | | | | | | | | | | | | | | | | | | | | | | | |

Arbeitsgruppe NFP ©

Identifying the infertile time at the beginning of the cycle and after ovulation

» **Annette W. is a 38-year-old geriatric nurse and mother of two children. This is her fifth cycle using Sensiplan.**

Trainings 19a and 19b are two successive cycles.
Annette W. observed a temperature shift in her previous cycle.

1. Identify the last infertile day at the beginning of the cycle and mark the first fertile day with "F."

2. Identify the shift in the cervical mucus sign.

3. Are there any disturbances or special circumstances?

4. Identify the earliest first higher temperature reading and enter this in the column on the right.

5. Identify the beginning of the infertile time after ovulation.

SENSIPLAN ®

Cycle-no*   5

Temperature taken   R X
   V
   O

Earliest first higher temperature reading in the previous cycles

   1 4

Minus 8

Earliest first higher temperature reading in this cycle

Do you intend to become pregnant in the next cycle?

yes
no X
undecided

Malteser
...weil Nähe zählt.

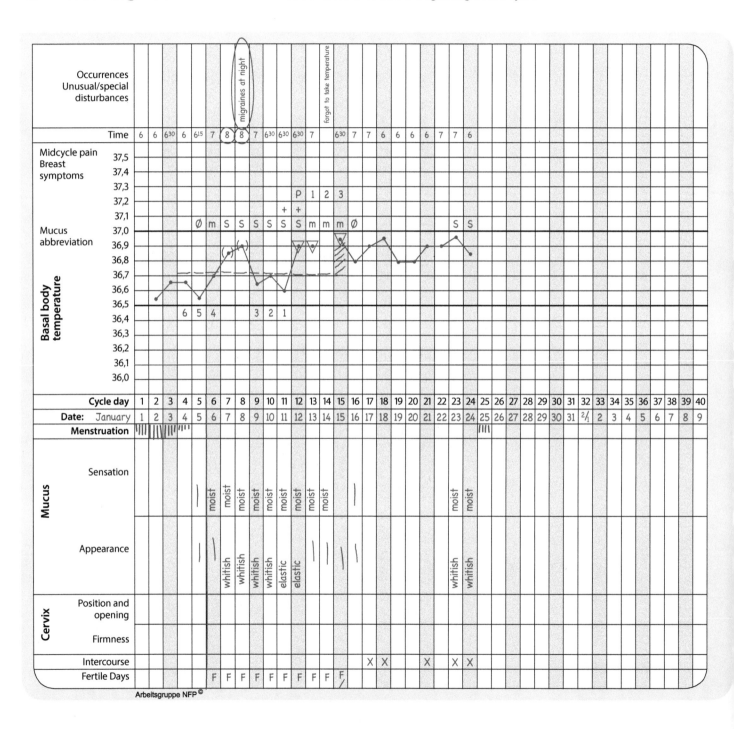

Identifying the infertile time at the beginning of the cycle and after ovulation

A temperature shift was observed in the previous cycle.

1. The infertile time at the beginning of the cycle was identified using the 5-Day Rule in double check with the cervical mucus sign. The last infertile day is cycle day 5.

2. The shift of the cervical mucus sign is on cycle day 12.

3. The late temperature measurement time on cycle days 7 and 8, and the migraine on cycle day 8, are disturbances. They are put in brackets and not taken into account when counting the six lower temperatures.

4. The earliest first higher temperature reading is on cycle day 12.

5. The infertile time after ovulation begins on the evening of cycle day 15.

®

Cycle-no* | 5

Temperature taken
R | X
V |
O |

Earliest first higher temperature reading in the previous cycles
1 | 4

Minus 8

Earliest first higher temperature reading in this cycle
1 | 2

Do you intend to become pregnant in the next cycle?

yes |
no | X
undecided |

Malteser
...weil Nähe zählt.

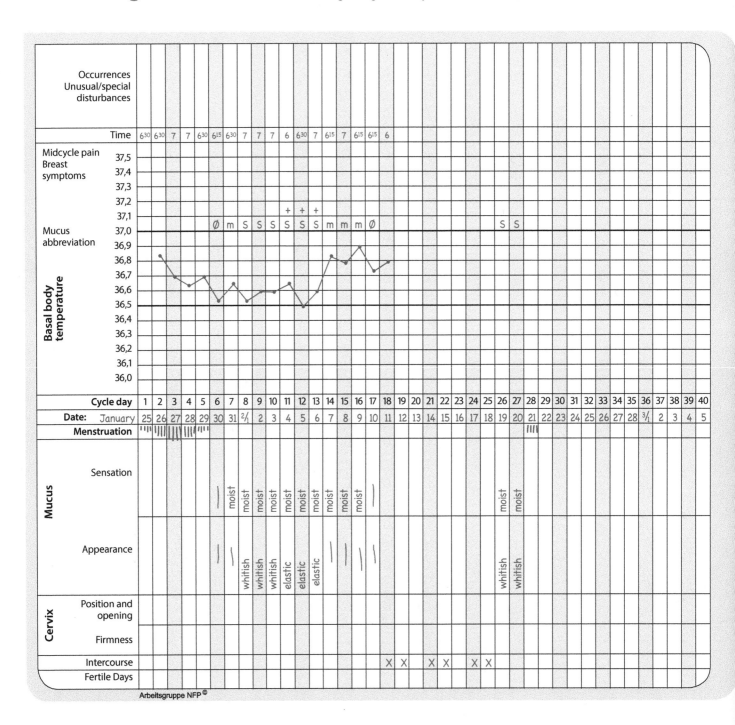

Occurrences Unusual/special disturbances

Time: 6³⁰ | 6³⁰ | 7 | 7 | 6³⁰ | 6¹⁵ | 6³⁰ | 7 | 7 | 7 | 6 | 6³⁰ | 7 | 6¹⁵ | 7 | 6¹⁵ | 6¹⁵ | 6

Midcycle pain / Breast symptoms

Mucus abbreviation (at 37,1 row): + + +
Mucus abbreviation (at 37,0 row): Ø m S S S S S S m m m Ø ... S S

Basal body temperature: 37,5 / 37,4 / 37,3 / 37,2 / 37,1 / 37,0 / 36,9 / 36,8 / 36,7 / 36,6 / 36,5 / 36,4 / 36,3 / 36,2 / 36,1 / 36,0

Cycle day	1	2	3	4	5	6	7	8	9	10	11	12	13	14	15	16	17	18	19	20	21	22	23	24	25	26	27	28	29	30	31	32	33	34	35	36	37	38	39	40
Date: January	25	26	27	28	29	30	31	²/₁	2	3	4	5	6	7	8	9	10	11	12	13	14	15	16	17	18	19	20	21	22	23	24	25	26	27	28	³/₁	2	3	4	5

Menstruation: (marked days 1–5, and days 27–28)

Mucus

Sensation: moist, moist, moist, moist, moist, moist, moist, moist, moist, moist ... moist, moist

Appearance: whitish, whitish, whitish, elastic, elastic, elastic ... whitish, whitish

Cervix — Position and opening / Firmness

Intercourse: X X X X X X

Fertile Days

Arbeitsgruppe NFP ©

Identifying the infertile time at the beginning of the cycle and after ovulation

Cycle-no*	6

Temperature taken	R	X
	V	
	O	

Earliest first higher temperature reading in the previous cycles

Minus 8

Earliest first higher temperature reading in this cycle

Do you intend to become pregnant in the next cycle?

yes

no X

undecided

✳ Malteser

...weil Nähe zählt.

» **This is Annette W.'s 6th cycle using Sensiplan.**

1. Identify the last infertile day at the beginning of the cycle and mark the first fertile day with "F."

2. Identify the shift in the cervical mucus sign.

3. Are there any disturbances or special circumstances?

4. Identify the earliest first higher temperature reading and enter this in the column on the right.

5. Identify the beginning of the infertile time after ovulation.

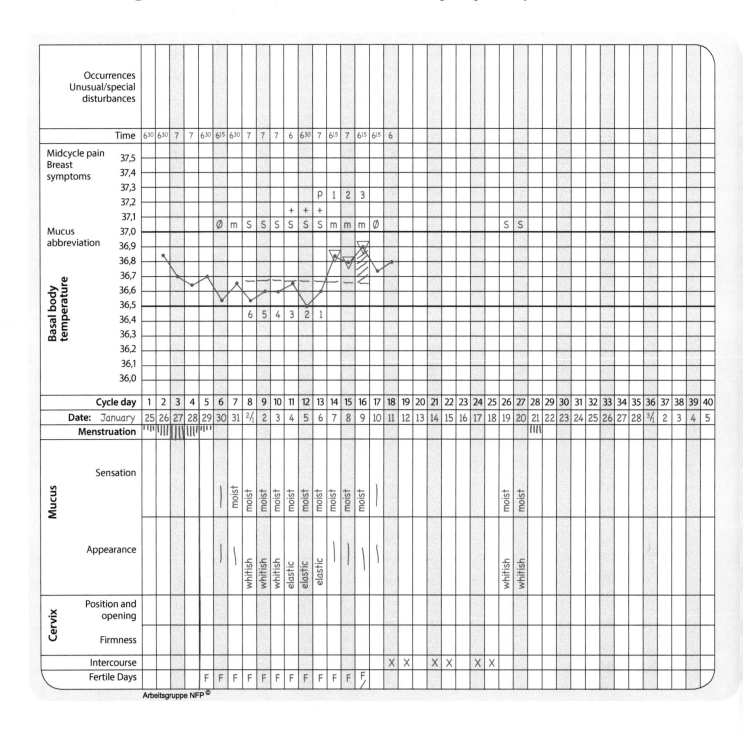

Arbeitsgruppe NFP ©

®

Cycle-no* | | 6 |

Temperature taken   R [X]
V [ ]
O [ ]

Earliest first higher temperature reading in the previous cycles | 1 | 2 |

Minus 8 | 4 |

Earliest first higher temperature reading in this cycle | 1 | 4 |

Do you intend to become pregnant in the next cycle?

yes [ ]
no [X]
undecided [ ]

✳ Malteser
...weil Nähe zählt.

Identifying the infertile time at the beginning of the cycle and after ovulation

1. Because the first higher temperature reading in a previous cycle was on cycle day 12, the infertile time at the beginning of the cycle is no longer identified using the 5-Day Rule (day 12 – day 8 = day 4, which is earlier than the 5-Day Rule). The Minus-8 Rule in double check with the cervical mucus sign shows the last infertile day as cycle day 4.

2. The shift of the cervical mucus sign is on cycle day 13.

3. No disturbances or special circumstances are recorded.

4. The earliest first higher temperature reading is on cycle day 14.

5. The infertile time after ovulation begins on the evening of cycle day 16.

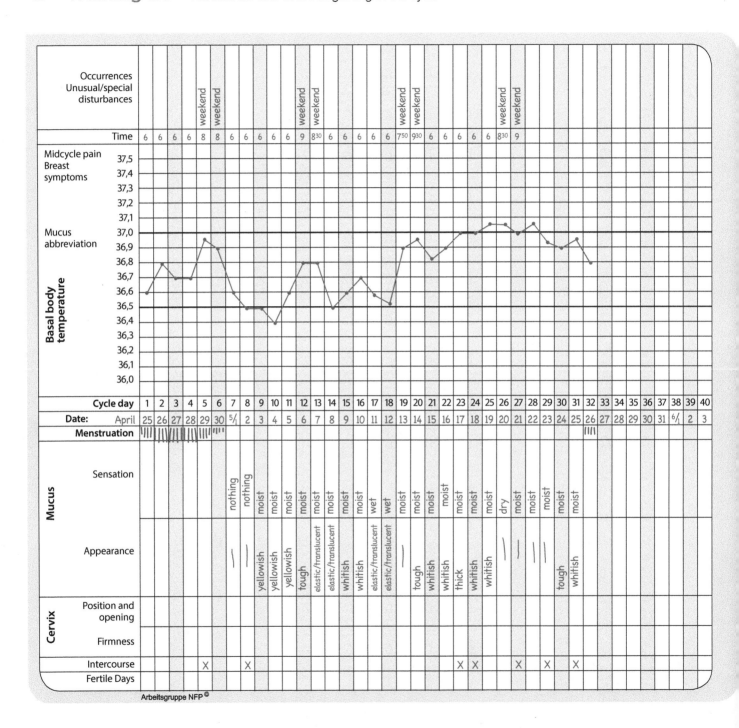

Occurrences Unusual/special disturbances					weekend	weekend						weekend	weekend					weekend	weekend						weekend	weekend															
Time	6	6	6	6	8	8	6	6	6	6	6	9	8³⁰	6	6	6	6	6	7⁵⁰	9³⁰	6	6	6	6	6	8³⁰	9														

Midcycle pain / Breast symptoms — Mucus abbreviation

Basal body temperature: 37,5 · 37,4 · 37,3 · 37,2 · 37,1 · 37,0 · 36,9 · 36,8 · 36,7 · 36,6 · 36,5 · 36,4 · 36,3 · 36,2 · 36,1 · 36,0

Cycle day	1	2	3	4	5	6	7	8	9	10	11	12	13	14	15	16	17	18	19	20	21	22	23	24	25	26	27	28	29	30	31	32	33	34	35	36	37	38	39	40
Date: April	25	26	27	28	29	30	5/1	2	3	4	5	6	7	8	9	10	11	12	13	14	15	16	17	18	19	20	21	22	23	24	25	26	27	28	29	30	31	6/1	2	3

Menstruation (cycle days 1–6, and days 31–32)

Mucus – Sensation: (7) nothing, (8) nothing, (9) moist, (10) moist, (11) moist, (12) moist, (13) moist, (14) moist, (15) moist, (16) moist, (17) wet, (18) wet, (19) moist, (20) moist, (21) moist, (22) moist, (23) moist, (24) moist, (25) moist, (26) dry, (27) moist, (28) moist, (29) moist, (30) moist, (31) moist

Mucus – Appearance: (7) \ , (9) yellowish, (10) yellowish, (11) yellowish, (12) tough, (13) elastic/translucent, (14) elastic/translucent, (15) whitish, (16) whitish, (17) elastic/translucent, (18) elastic/translucent, (19)), (20) tough, (21) whitish, (22) whitish, (23) thick, (24) whitish, (25) whitish, (26) \, (27) \, (28) \ \, (30) tough, (31) whitish

Cervix – Position and opening / **Firmness**

Intercourse: day 4 X, day 8 X, day 23 X, day 24 X, day 26 X, day 28 X, day 30 X

Fertile Days

Arbeitsgruppe NFP ©

Identifying the infertile time at the beginning of the cycle and after ovulation

» **Marta M. is a 25-year-old designer.**

A temperature shift was observed in the previous cycle.

1. Identify the last infertile day at the beginning of the cycle and mark the first fertile day with "F."

2. Identify the shift in the cervical mucus sign.

3. Are there any disturbances or special circumstances?

4. Identify the earliest first higher temperature reading and enter this in the column on the right.

5. Identify the beginning of the infertile time after ovulation.

---

sensiplan ®

Cycle-no* | 1 | 3 |

Temperature taken   R | X |
                       V | |
                       O | |

Earliest first higher temperature reading in the previous cycles | 1 | 5 |

Minus 8

Earliest first higher temperature reading in this cycle

Do you intend to become pregnant in the next cycle?

yes

no | X |

undecided

✳ **Malteser**
...weil Nähe zählt.

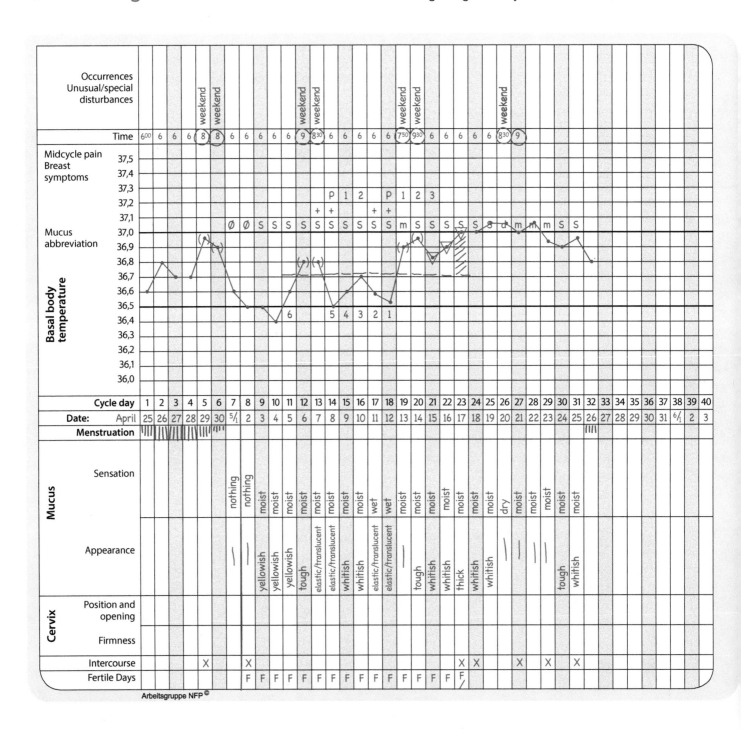

Arbeitsgruppe NFP ©

Identifying the infertile time at the beginning of the cycle and after ovulation

®

| Cycle-no* | 1 | 3 |

Temperature taken

R [X]

V [ ]

O [ ]

Earliest first higher temperature reading in the previous cycles

| 1 | 5 |

Minus 8 | 7 |

Earliest first higher temperature reading in this cycle

| 2 | 1 |

Do you intend to become pregnant in the next cycle?

yes [ ]

no [X]

undecided [ ]

❋ Malteser

...weil Nähe zählt.

1. There are two shifts in the cervical mucus sign – on cycle days 14 and 18.

2. The infertile time at the beginning of the cycle was identified using the Minus-8 Rule in double check with the cervical mucus sign. The last infertile day is cycle day 7.

3. It appears that taking temperatures later than usual on the weekends affects Marta M.'s temperature measurements on cycle days 5, 6, 12, 13, 19, 20, 26, and 27 and are counted as distubances.

4. The earliest first higher temperature reading is on cycle day 21.

5. The infertile time after ovulation begins on the evening of cycle day 23.

Note:
*   The mucus shift on cycle day 18 is used for the double check because the best quality cervical mucus is present again before the temperature evaluation has been completed.

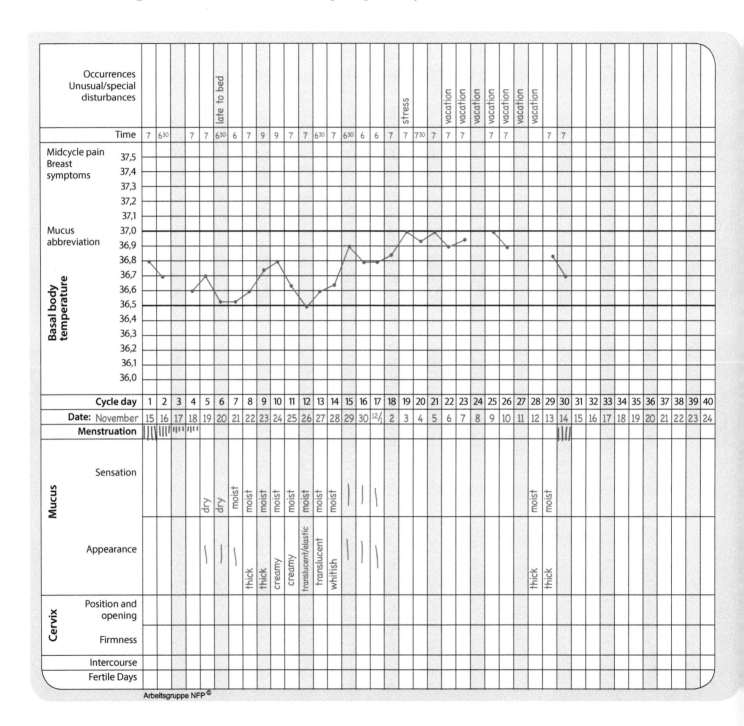

Identifying the infertile time at the beginning of the cycle and after ovulation

» **Nala O. is a 29-year-old accountant. She has been using Sensiplan for over a year.**

A temperature shift was observed in the previous cycle.

1. Enter the cervical mucus abbreviations and identify the shift in the cervical mucus sign.

2. Identify the last infertile day at the beginning of the cycle and mark the first fertile day with "F."

3. Are there any disturbances or special circumstances?

4. Identify the earliest first higher temperature reading and enter this in the column on the right.

5. Identify the beginning of the infertile time after ovulation.

SENSIPLAN ®

Cycle-no*   1 5

Temperature taken
R
V X
O

Earliest first higher temperature reading in the previous cycles

1 6

Minus 8

Earliest first higher temperature reading in this cycle

Do you intend to become pregnant in the next cycle?

yes
no
undecided X

✳ **Malteser**
...weil Nähe zählt.

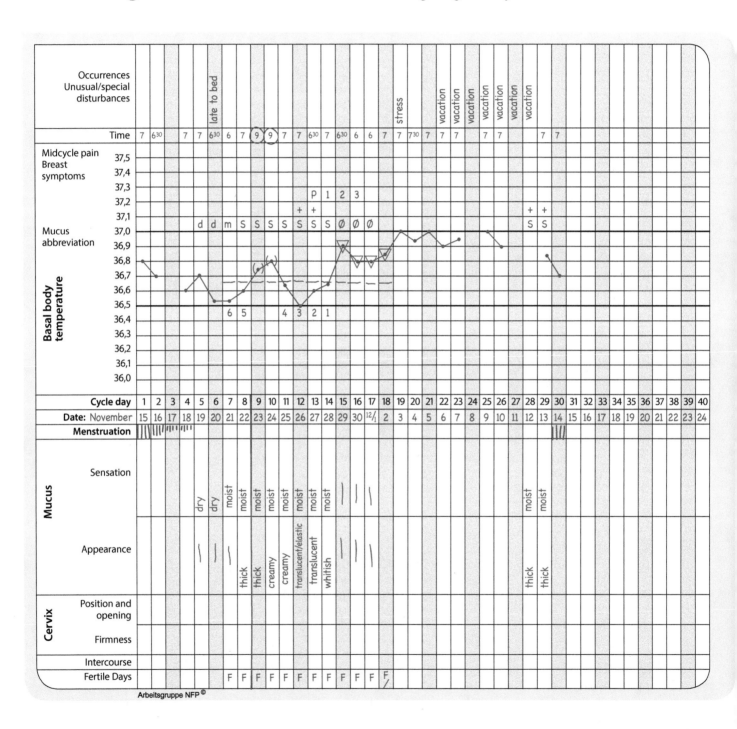

Arbeitsgruppe NFP ©

Identifying the infertile time at the beginning of the cycle and after ovulation

Cycle-no*		1	5

Temperature taken	R	
	V	X
	O	

Earliest first higher temperature reading in the previous cycles

	1	6

Minus 8		8

Earliest first higher temperature reading in this cycle

	1	5

Do you intend to become pregnant in the next cycle?

yes	
no	
undecided	X

1. The shift of the cervical mucus sign is on cycle day 13.

2. The infertile time at the beginning of the cycle is identified using the Minus-8 Rule in double check with the cervical mucus sign. The last infertile day at the beginning of the cycle is cycle day 6.

3. On cycle day 6, "late to bed" did not affect the temperature measurement and was not counted as a disturbance. However, on cycle days 9 and 10, the late temperature measurement did cause a disturbance and is put in brackets. These values are not taken into account when counting the six lower temperatures.

4. The earliest first higher temperature reading is on cycle day 15, one day earlier than any previous earliest first higher temperature reading. Enter this in the column on the right.

5. The infertile time after ovulation begins on the evening of cycle day 18.

Note:
- The temperature shift is evaluated using the first exception to the rule.

✳ Malteser
...weil Nähe zählt.

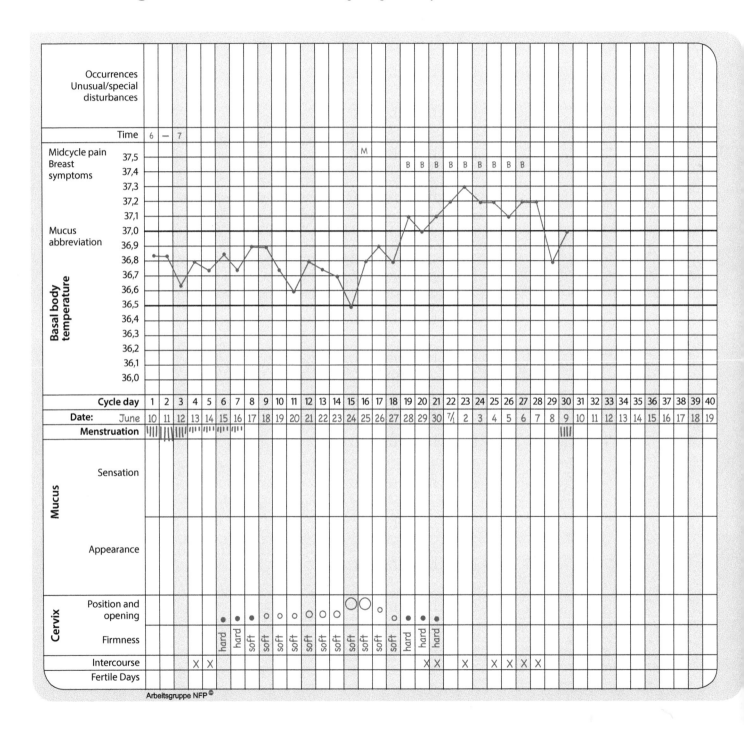

Identifying the infertile time at the beginning of the cycle and after ovulation

» Renate S. is 41 years old and has been using Sensiplan for several years. Because she had several days of bleeding in the beginning of her cycle, and she typically observes small amounts of cervical mucus throughout her cycle, she identifies the beginning and end of the fertile time using the cervix sign.

Trainings 22a and 22b are two successive cycles.
Renate S. did not observe a temperature shift in the previous cycle.

1. Identify the last infertile day at the beginning of the cycle and mark the first fertile day with "F."

2. Are there any disturbances or special circumstances?

3. Identify the earliest first higher temperature reading and enter this in the column on the right.

4. Identify the beginning of the infertile time after ovulation.

SENSIPLAN ®

Cycle-no* | 6 | 8

Temperature taken R | X
V |
O |

Earliest first higher temperature reading in the previous cycles | 1 | 5

Minus 8

Earliest first higher temperature reading in this cycle

Do you intend to become pregnant in the next cycle?

yes
no | X
undecided

✠ Malteser
...weil Nähe zählt.

Training 22a – Solution
The infertile time at the beginning of the cycle

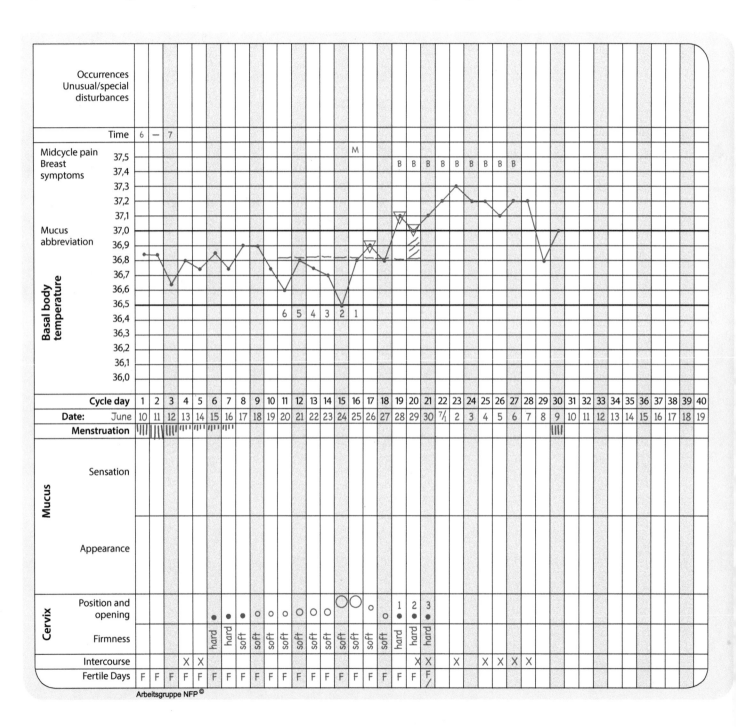

Arbeitsgruppe NFP ©

Identifying the infertile time at the beginning of the cycle and after ovulation

Cycle-no* 6 8

Temperature taken
R X
V
O

Earliest first higher temperature reading in the previous cycles
1 5

Minus 8

Earliest first higher temperature reading in this cycle
1 7

Do you intend to become pregnant in the next cycle?
yes
no X
undecided

Malteser
...weil Nähe zählt.

1. Because Renate S. did not measure her temperature in the previous cycle, she cannot assume any infertile days at the beginning of the current cycle.

2. No disturbances or special circumstances are recorded.

3. The earliest first higher temperature reading is on cycle day 17.

4. The infertile time after ovulation begins on the evening of cycle day 21 using a double check with the cervix sign.

Note:
- The temperature shift is evaluated using the second exception to the rule.

Comment: Although Renate S. recorded that she does not intend to become pregnant this cycle, she recorded intercourse during the fertile time on cycle days 4, 5, and 20.

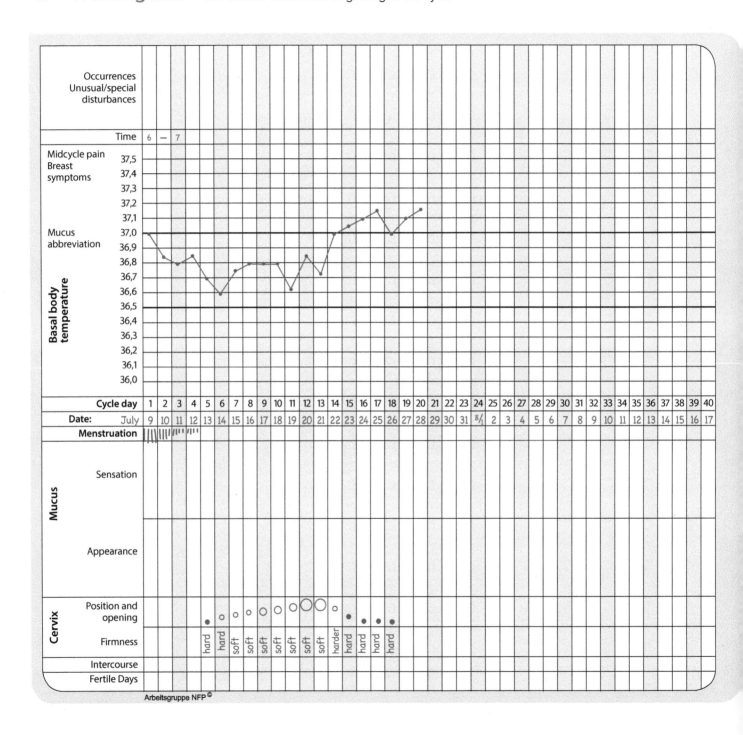

| Occurrences Unusual/special disturbances | | | | | | | | | | | | | | | | | | | | | | | | | | | | | | | | | | | | | | | |

| Time | 6 — 7 |

Midcycle pain Breast symptoms

Mucus abbreviation

Basal body temperature

| 37,5 |
| 37,4 |
| 37,3 |
| 37,2 |
| 37,1 |
| 37,0 |
| 36,9 |
| 36,8 |
| 36,7 |
| 36,6 |
| 36,5 |
| 36,4 |
| 36,3 |
| 36,2 |
| 36,1 |
| 36,0 |

Cycle day	1	2	3	4	5	6	7	8	9	10	11	12	13	14	15	16	17	18	19	20	21	22	23	24	25	26	27	28	29	30	31	32	33	34	35	36	37	38	39	40
Date: July	9	10	11	12	13	14	15	16	17	18	19	20	21	22	23	24	25	26	27	28	29	30	31	8/1	2	3	4	5	6	7	8	9	10	11	12	13	14	15	16	17
Menstruation	‖‖‖‖‖‖ʼʼ																																							

Mucus

| Sensation | | | | | | | | | | | | | | | | | | | | | | | | | | | | | | | | | | | | | | | | |
| Appearance | | | | | | | | | | | | | | | | | | | | | | | | | | | | | | | | | | | | | | | | |

Cervix

Position and opening				●	○	○	○	○	○	○	○	○	○	●	●	●	●																							
Firmness				hard	hard	soft	soft	soft	soft	soft	soft	soft	harder	hard	hard	hard	hard																							
Intercourse																																								
Fertile Days																																								

Arbeitsgruppe NFP ©

sensiPLAN ®

Cycle-no* 6 9

**Temperature
taken** R X

V

O

Earliest first higher
temperature reading
in the previous cycles

1 5

Minus 8

Earliest first higher
temperature
reading in
this cycle

Do you intend to
become pregnant
in the next cycle?

yes

no X

undecided

✳ **Malteser**
...weil Nähe zählt.

Identifying the infertile time at the beginning of the cycle and after ovulation

» **This is Renate S.'s 69th cycle chart.**

1. Identify the last infertile day at the beginning of the cycle and mark the first fertile day with "F."

2. Are there any disturbances or special circumstances?

3. Identify the earliest first higher temperature reading and enter this in the column on the right.

4. Identify the beginning of the infertile time after ovulation.

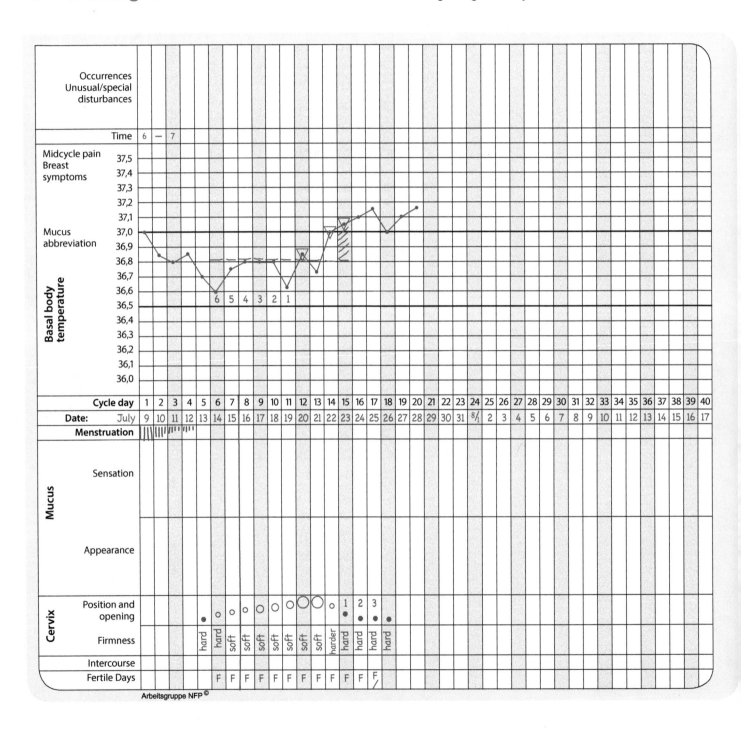

Occurrences Unusual/special disturbances																																										
Time	6	—	7																																							

Cycle day 1 2 3 4 5 6 7 8 9 10 11 12 13 14 15 16 17 18 19 20 21 22 23 24 25 26 27 28 29 30 31 32 33 34 35 36 37 38 39 40

Date: July 9 10 11 12 13 14 15 16 17 18 19 20 21 22 23 24 25 26 27 28 29 30 31 8/1 2 3 4 5 6 7 8 9 10 11 12 13 14 15 16 17

Menstruation |||||| ////// ///

Cervix																	
Position and opening			•	○	○	○	○	○	○	○ ○	○	○	1 •	2 •	3 •	•	
Firmness			hard	hard	soft	soft	soft	soft	soft	soft	soft	harder	hard	hard	hard	hard	

Intercourse

Fertile Days F F F F F F F F F F F F F/

Arbeitsgruppe NFP ©

Identifying the infertile time at the beginning of the cycle and after ovulation

Cycle-no*	6 9

Temperature taken	R	X
	V	
	O	

Earliest first higher
temperature reading
in the previous cycles

| 1 | 5 |

Minus 8   7

Earliest first higher
temperature
reading in
this cycle   1 2

Do you intend to
become pregnant
in the next cycle?

yes ☐

no X

undecided ☐

Malteser
...weil Nähe zählt.

1. The infertile time at the beginning of the cycle is identified using the Minus-8 Rule in double check with the cervix sign. The last infertile day is cycle day 5.

2. No disturbances or special circumstances are recorded.

3. The earliest first higher temperature reading is on cycle day 12. Therefore, for all future charts, the earliest first higher temperature reading in the previous cycles must be changed to 12. Enter this in the column on the right.

4. The infertile time after ovulation begins on the evening of cycle day 17.

Note:
- The temperature shift is evaluated using the second exception to the rule.

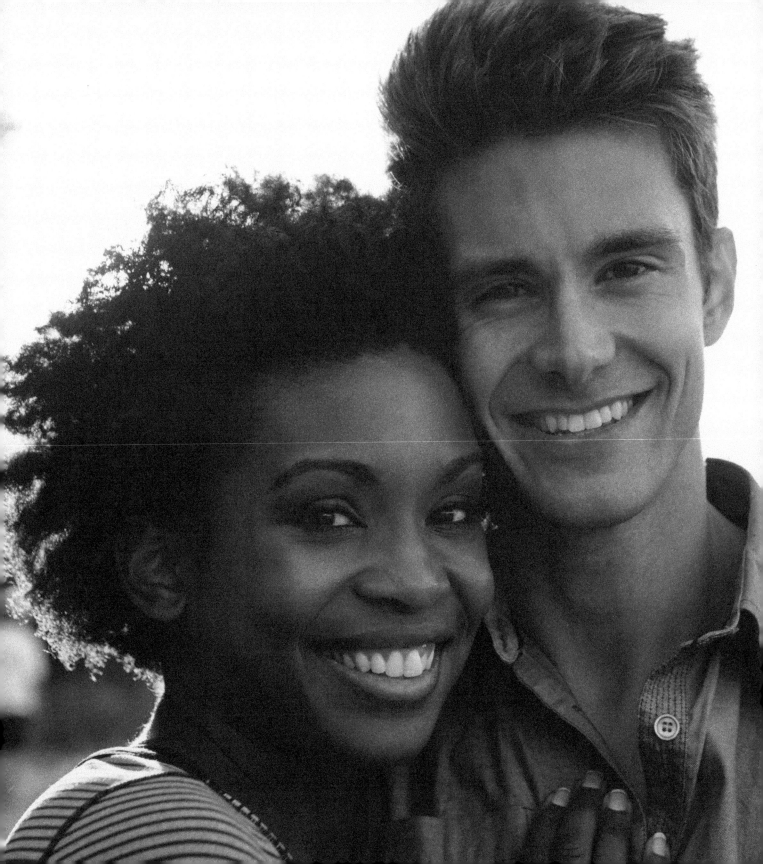

Chapter 4:

Special life circumstances and cycle patterns

Sensiplan is a family planning method that can be used by women throughout their fertile years and into perimenopause. This chapter has a range of sample cycles from women in various phases of life, with brief explanations and several examples of the changes that may be observed during those phases of life.

Cycle patterns

Many people believe a normal cycle length is 28 days long. However, for most women, the length of a cycle can naturally fluctuate from cycle to cycle. Although every woman has her own individual cycle pattern, cycles between 25 and 35 days are considered regular. Each cycle consists of two phases: the follicular phase (beginning of cycle up to ovulation) and the luteal phase (ovulation through the end of the cycle). It is the follicular phase that is responsible for the fluctuation of the cycle length. In long cycles, the follicular phase is extended, and ovulation occurs later than in shorter cycles.

Cycles with a short luteal phase

Typically the luteal phase is stable in length and begins about 10-16 days before menstruation begins. If this phase is shorter than ten days, it is referred to as a short luteal phase. In these cycles, the chance of pregnancy is reduced because the luteal phase is not long enough for a fertilized egg to implant in the lining of the uterus.

Monophasic cycles

Cycles where there is no ovulation (and no temperature shift), are called monophasic cycles. During these cycles, bleeding may occur; however, the user must consider herself fertile until she has confirmed ovulation using the double check method. The fertile phase continues until a temperature shift can be identified in double check with the cervical mucus or cervix position sign.

Cycle patterns are closely related to a woman's natural life and maturity processes. Although women with varying cycle patterns can have normal fertility, some women may have a more difficult time getting pregnant. Irregular cycle lengths, cycles with a short luteal phase, and monophasic cycles are common during life phases where there are hormonal changes. This includes young women in the first years after the onset of puberty, after pregnancy, during breastfeeding, at the beginning of perimenopause, and after discontinuing hormonal contraceptives.

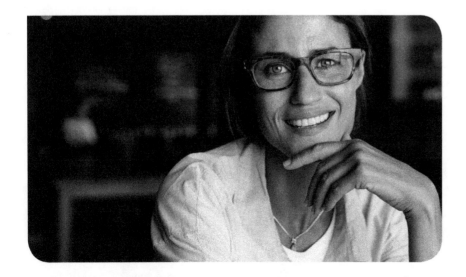

Special life circumstances

Trying to conceive

The greatest chance of conceiving a pregnancy is when intercourse occurs:

• On days with the best quality cervical mucus, and the days directly following this, up to and including the day with the first higher temperature reading

• On days where the cervix is open, soft, and high

• On days where there is mid-cycle pain or mid-cycle bleeding

Identifying a pregnancy:
If the temperature shift remains elevated for more than 18 days and there has been no bleeding, pregnancy is likely.

Rule:
Date of the first higher temperature reading minus 7 days, minus 3 months, plus 1 year = anticipated due date.

Example:
--first higher temperature reading 7/13/2019
--minus 7 days = 7/6/19
--minus 3 months = 4/6/19
--plus 1 year = 4/6/20 is the anticipated due date

7/13/2019		7/6/2019		4/6/2019
− 7 Days		− 3 Months		+ 1 Year
= **7/6/2019**		= **4/6/2019**		= 4/6/2020

After giving birth and during breastfeeding

After giving birth and during breastfeeding observing your body can provide valuable information about the return of fertility and the need for family planning.

Until the first temperature shift is evaluated, special rules apply during breastfeeding, which is explained in detail in *Natural & Safe: The Handbook* in the chapter entitled, "Breastfeeding."

To evaluate the first temperature shift after giving birth, an additional higher temperature measurement (above the cover line) is required.

Perimenopause

Senisplan can be used by women during perimenopause and may allow them to understand better their waning fertility and how it relates to family planning. There are several special rules for this phase that are discussed in detail in *Natural & Safe: The Handbook* in the chapter entitled, "Perimenopause."

After discontinuing hormonal contraceptives

After discontinuing hormonal contraceptives, women can use Sensiplan to recognize the return to normal cycle patterns by using cervical mucus and temperature signs.

• If you stop hormonal contraception and do not begin to bleed during the first week, consider yourself infertile for the first 7 days after discontinuing your hormonal contraception. Your fertility will begin on day 8.

• If you have a menstrual bleed before that time, consider yourself infertile for the first 5 days of the cycle. Your fertility will begin on day 6.

• To evaluate the temperature shift in the first cycle after discontinuing hormonal contraception, one additional higher temperature measurement is required. The additional temperature measurement must be above the cover line but does not have to be 0.2 °C above. The infertile time begins on the evening of the day with the fourth higher temperature reading or the day when the cervical mucus sign has been completed, whichever comes last.

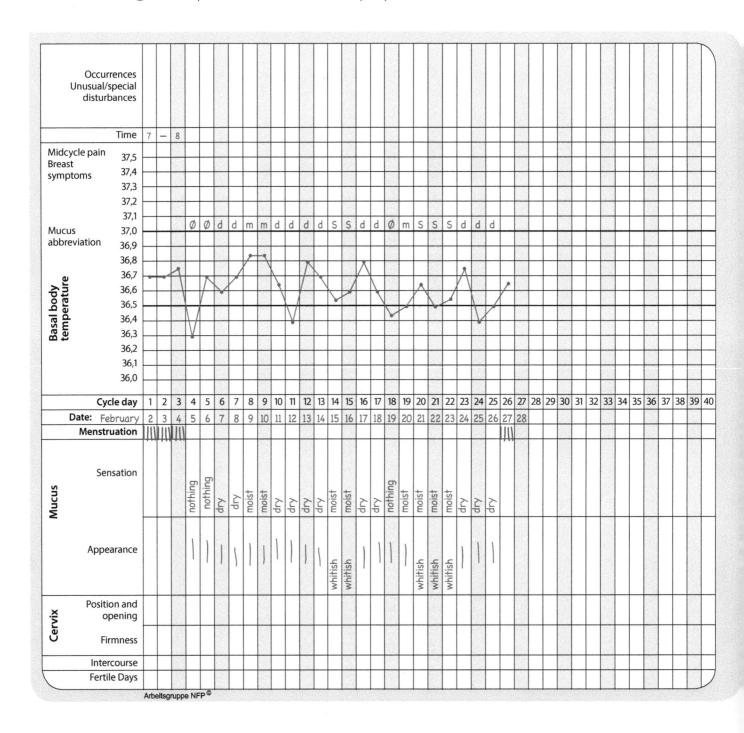

Arbeitsgruppe NFP ©

SENSIPLAN ®

Cycle-no* 5

Temperature taken
R X
V
O

Earliest first higher temperature reading in the previous cycles

2 2

Minus 8

Earliest first higher temperature reading in this cycle

Do you intend to become pregnant in the next cycle?

yes

no

undecided

✠ **Malteser**
...weil Nähe zählt.

Monophasic cycles

» Rachel P. is a 15-year-old student. She is learning how to observe her body's signs of ovulation using Sensiplan.

There was a temperature shift in the previous cycle.

1. Identify the beginning and end of the fertile time and mark this phase with "F."

2. Are there any disturbances or special circumstances?

3. What do you notice?

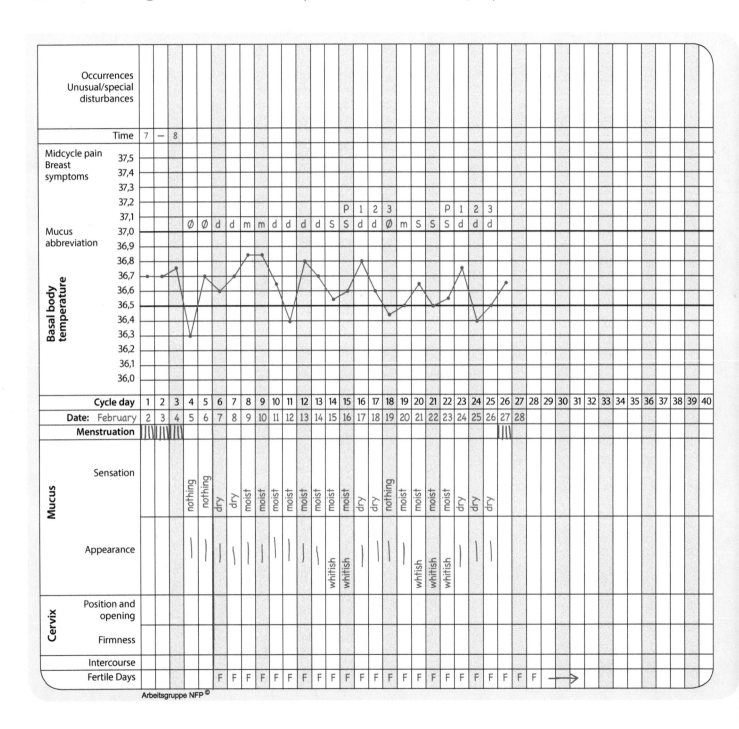

Arbeitsgruppe NFP ©

®

Cycle-no* | | 5

Temperature taken

R [X]

V [ ]

O [ ]

Earliest first higher temperature reading in the previous cycles

[2] [2]

Minus 8

[⟋]

Earliest first higher temperature reading in this cycle

[⟋]

Do you intend to become pregnant in the next cycle?

yes [ ]

no [ ]

undecided [ ]

![Malteser logo] **Malteser**
...weil Nähe zählt.

Monophasic cycles

1. The infertile time at the beginning of the cycle is identified using the 5-Day Rule in double check with the cervical mucus sign. The last infertile day is cycle day 5. Since there is no confirmed temperature shift in this cycle, ovulation cannot be confirmed. Therefore, in the beginning of the next cycle, no infertile days can be assumed, and Rachel P. will mark "F" beginning on cycle day 1.

2. No disturbances or special circumstances are recorded. However, there are two shifts in the cervical mucus sign.

3. This cycle chart is an example of a typical monophasic cycle. Monophasic cycles are common in puberty and perimenopause.

Cycle day	1	2	3	4	5	6	7	8	9	10	11	12	13	14	15	16	17	18	19	20	21	22	23	24	25	26	27	28	29	30	31	32	33	34	35	36	37	38	39	40
Occurrences Unusual/special disturbances		lots of stress	lots of stress	lots of stress	lots of stress	lots of stress	lots of stress	lots of stress	lots of stress	lots of stress	lots of stress				cold																									
Time	7																																							
Midcycle pain / Breast symptoms																							M	M			B	B	B	B	B					B	B			
Mucus abbreviation					d	d	d	d	d	S	d	d	d	d	Ø	S	S	d	d	d	d	S	S	S	S	d	d	d	d	d	d	d	d	d	S	S	S			
Date: August	7	8	9	10	11	12	13	14	15	16	17	18	19	20	21	22	23	24	25	26	27	28	29	30	31	9/1	2	3	4	5	6	7	8	9	10	11	12	13	14	15
Menstruation	‖	‖	‖	‖	‖	‖	‖																													‖	‖	‖	‖	‖

Basal body temperature (°C): scale 36,0 – 37,5

Cycle day	Sensation	Appearance	Cervix Position/opening	Firmness
5	dry	ǀ	●	hard
6	dry	ǀ	●	hard
7	dry	ǀ	●	hard
8	dry	ǀ	●	hard
9	moist	creamy	●	hard
10	dry	ǀ	●	hard
11	dry	ǀ	●	hard
12	dry	ǀ	●	hard
13	dry	ǀ	●	hard
14	dry	ǀ	●	hard
15	ǀ		●	hard
16	moist	elastic	●	softer
17	moist	creamy	●	softer
18	dry	ǀ	●	hard
19	dry	ǀ	●	hard
20	dry	ǀ	●	hard
21	dry		○	softer
22	moist	thick	○	soft
23	wet	elastic	○	soft
24	wet	elastic	○	soft
25	moist	tough	○	harder
26	dry	ǀ	●	hard
27	dry	ǀ	●	hard
28	dry	ǀ	●	hard
29	dry	ǀ	●	hard
30	dry	ǀ	●	hard
31	dry	ǀ	●	hard
32	dry	ǀ	●	hard
33	dry	ǀ	●	hard
34	moist	tough	○	softer
35	wet	translucent	○	softer
36	wet	reddish	○	

Intercourse —

Fertile Days —

Arbeitsgruppe NFP ©

Cycle-no*		1	6

Temperature taken	R	
	V	
	O	X

Earliest first higher temperature reading in the previous cycles

	1	5

Minus 8

Earliest first higher temperature reading in this cycle

Do you intend to become pregnant in the next cycle?

yes	
no	X
undecided	

Malteser
...weil Nähe zählt.

Prolonged follicular phase

» **Stephanie W. is a 30-year-old mother of one child; she is currently on maternity leave.**

There was a temperature shift in the previous cycle.

1. Identify the beginning and end of the fertile time and mark this phase with "F."

2. Are there any disturbances or special circumstances?

3. What do you notice?

Cycle day	1	2	3	4	5	6	7	8	9	10	11	12	13	14	15	16	17	18	19	20	21	22	23	24	25	26	27	28	29	30	31	32	33	34	35	36	37	38	39	40
Date: August	7	8	9	10	11	12	13	14	15	16	17	18	19	20	21	22	23	24	25	26	27	28	29	30	31	9/1	2	3	4	5	6	7	8	9	10	11	12	13	14	15

Occurrences / Unusual/special disturbances: "lots of stress" (cycle days 1–10); "cold" (circled, around cycle day 15)

Midcycle pain / Breast symptoms: M (day 23), M (day 24); B (days 27, 28, 29, 30, 31); B (days 36, 37)

Mucus abbreviation (P/+/numbers):
- P, 1, 2, 3 at days 17–20
- P, 1, 2, 3 at days 24–27
- + at day 18; + at days 23, 24; + at days 36, 37
- d d d d d d S d d d d Ø S S d d d d d S S S S d d d d d d d d t S S S (mucus letters across days 5–39)

Basal body temperature (°C, range 36,0–37,5): daily values plotted. Count-up numbers under curve: 6 5 4 3 2 1 (days 19–24). Temperature shift line at days 25–27.

	Sensation	Appearance	Position and opening	Firmness
Day 6	dry	|	•	hard
Day 7	dry	\	•	hard
Day 8	dry	|	•	hard
Day 9	dry	|	•	hard
Day 10	dry		•	hard
Day 11	moist	creamy	•	hard
Day 12	dry	|	•	hard
Day 13	dry	|	•	hard
Day 14	dry	|	•	hard
Day 15	dry	|	•	hard
Day 16				hard
Day 17	moist	elastic		softer
Day 18	moist	creamy	•	softer
Day 19	dry	|	1	hard
Day 20	dry	|	2	hard
Day 21	dry	|	3	hard
Day 22	dry		o	softer
Day 23	moist	thick	o	soft
Day 24	wet	elastic	o	soft
Day 25	wet	elastic	o	soft
Day 26	moist	tough	o	harder
Day 27	dry	|	1	hard
Day 28	dry	|	2	hard
Day 29	dry	|	3	hard
Day 30	dry	|	•	hard
Day 31	dry	|	•	hard
Day 32	dry	|	•	hard
Day 33	dry		•	hard
Day 34	dry		•	hard
Day 35	moist	tough	o	softer
Day 36	wet	translucent	o	softer
Day 37	wet	reddish		

Menstruation: days 1–5 (with tapering marks) and days 38–40 (next cycle)

Fertile Days (F): marked from cycle day 6 through cycle day 25 (F row shows F on days 6–24, with slash/end marker at day 25)

Arbeitsgruppe NFP ©

Prolonged follicular phase

Cycle-no* `1` `6`

Temperature taken
R `　`
V `　`
O `X`

Earliest first higher temperature reading in the previous cycles `1` `5`

Minus 8 `7`

Earliest first higher temperature reading in this cycle `2` `5`

Do you intend to become pregnant in the next cycle?
yes `　`
no `X`
undecided `　`

Malteser
...weil Nähe zählt.

1. The infertile time at the beginning of the cycle is identified using the Minus-8 Rule in double check with the cervical mucus sign. The last infertile day is cycle day 7. The infertile time after ovulation begins on the evening of cycle day 28.

2. On cycle day 15, a cold affected the temperature measurement and is counted as a disturbance. This value is put in brackets and not taken into account when evaluating the temperature shift.

3. This cycle chart is an example of a prolonged follicular phase. For Stephanie W., her cycle length is 37 days long which is caused by a delayed follicular phase of 24 days. The luteal phase is normal at 13 days. A possible cause of the prolonged follicular phase is the period of stress at the beginning of the cycle.

4. Because the beginning and end of the fertile time are evaluated using the cervical mucus sign and basal body temperature, it is not necessary to also include the evaluation of the cervix sign. A "triple check" is not necessary.

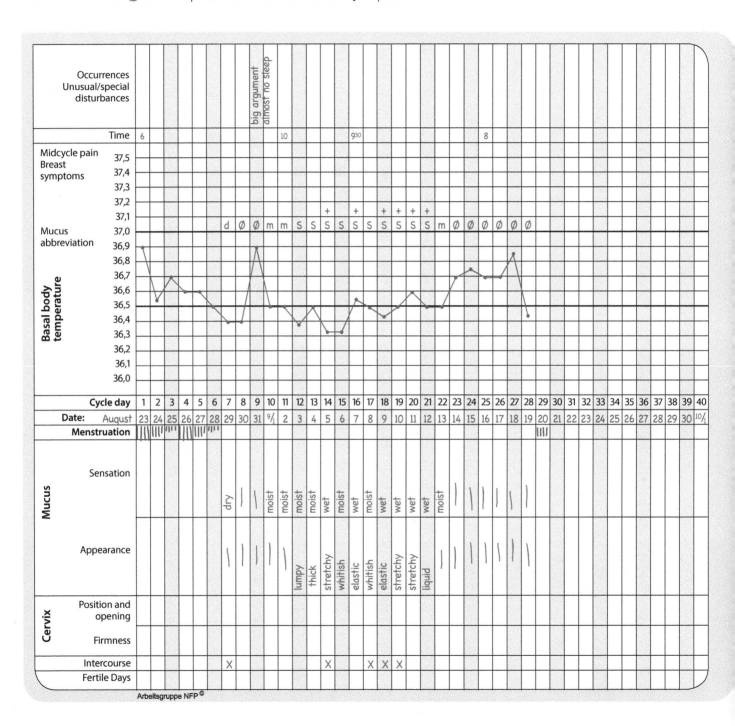

sensiplan ®

Cycle-no* | 1 | 4

Temperature taken
R |
V |
O | X

Earliest first higher temperature reading in the previous cycles

1 | 7

Minus 8

Earliest first higher temperature reading in this cycle

Do you intend to become pregnant in the next cycle?

yes | X
no |
undecided |

✠ Malteser
...weil Nähe zählt.

Short luteal phase

» Lydia G. is a 31-year-old nurse with no children. She has been trying to conceive for 6 months.

There was a temperature shift in the previous cycle.

1. Identify the beginning and end of the fertile time and mark this phase with "F."

2. Are there any disturbances or special circumstances?

3. What do you notice?

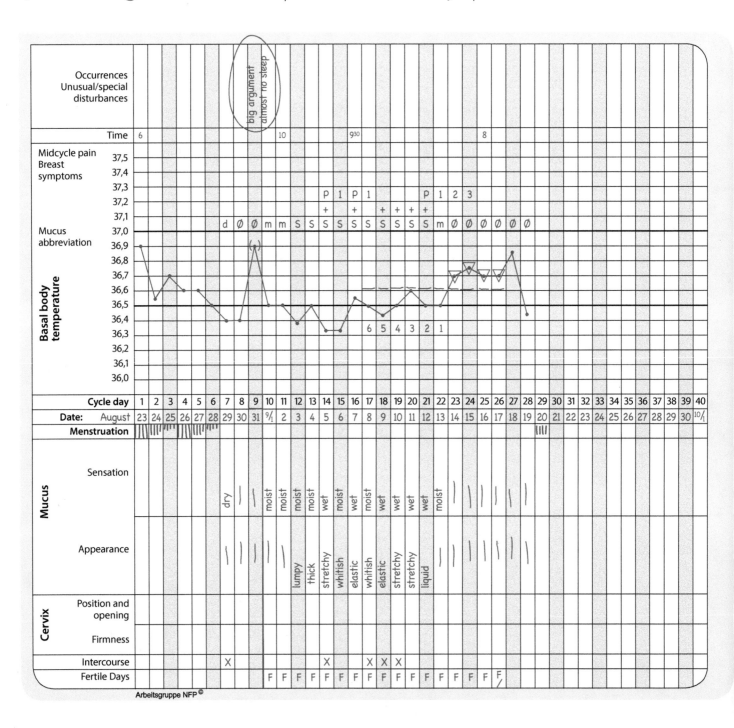

Arbeitsgruppe NFP ©

®

Cycle-no* | 1 | 4 |

Temperature taken

R ☐

V ☐

O ☒

Earliest first higher
temperature reading
in the previous cycles

| 1 | 7 |

Minus 8 | 9 |

Earliest first higher
temperature
reading in
this cycle | 2 | 3 |

Do you intend to
become pregnant
in the next cycle?

yes ☒

no ☐

undecided ☐

✳ Malteser
...weil Nähe zählt.

Short luteal phase

1. The infertile time at the beginning of the cycle is identified using the Minus-8 Rule in double check with the cervical mucus sign. The last infertile day is cycle day 9. The infertile time after ovulation begins on the evening of cycle day 26.

2. On cycle days 11 and 25, the late measuring times did not affect the temperature measurement and are not put in brackets. However, on cycle day 9, "big argument, almost no sleep" affected the temperature measurement and is put in brackets. This value is not taken into account in the temperature shift evaluation.

3. In this cycle, the temperature shift is only six days long, which shows a short luteal phase. This may be the reason why Lydia G. did not become pregnant in this cycle.

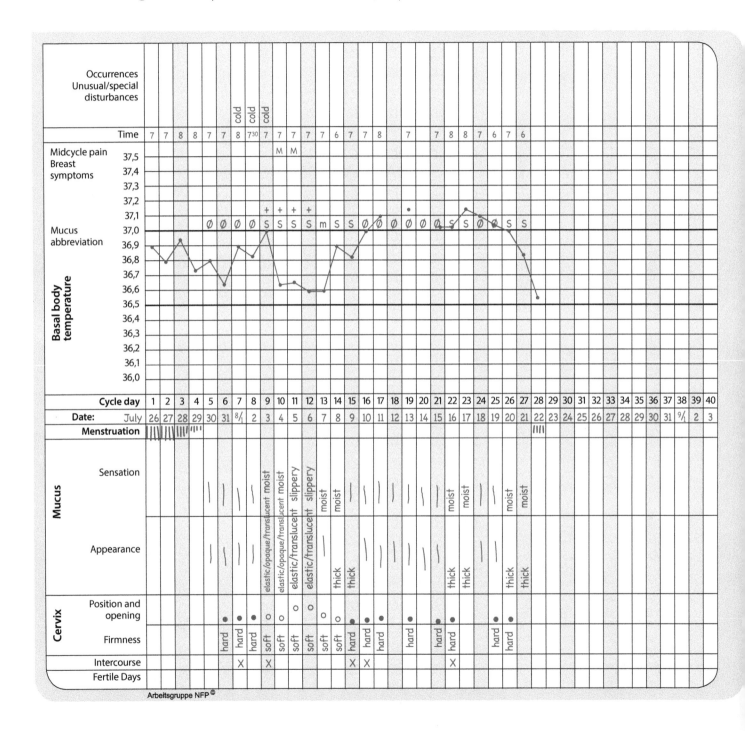

Arbeitsgruppe NFP ©

SENSIPLAN ®

Cycle-no*		1	7

Temperature taken

R X
V ☐
O ☐

Earliest first higher temperature reading in the previous cycles

	1	4

Minus 8 ☐☐

Earliest first higher temperature reading in this cycle ☐☐

Do you intend to become pregnant in the next cycle?

yes X
no ☐
undecided ☐

✠ Malteser
...weil Nähe zählt.

Trying to conceive

» **Cristina L. is 31 years old and has been trying to conceive for four cycles.**

Trainings 26a and 26b are two successive cycles.

There was a temperature shift in the previous cycle.

1. Identify the beginning and end of the fertile time and mark this phase with "F."

2. Are there any disturbances or special circumstances?

3. What do you notice?

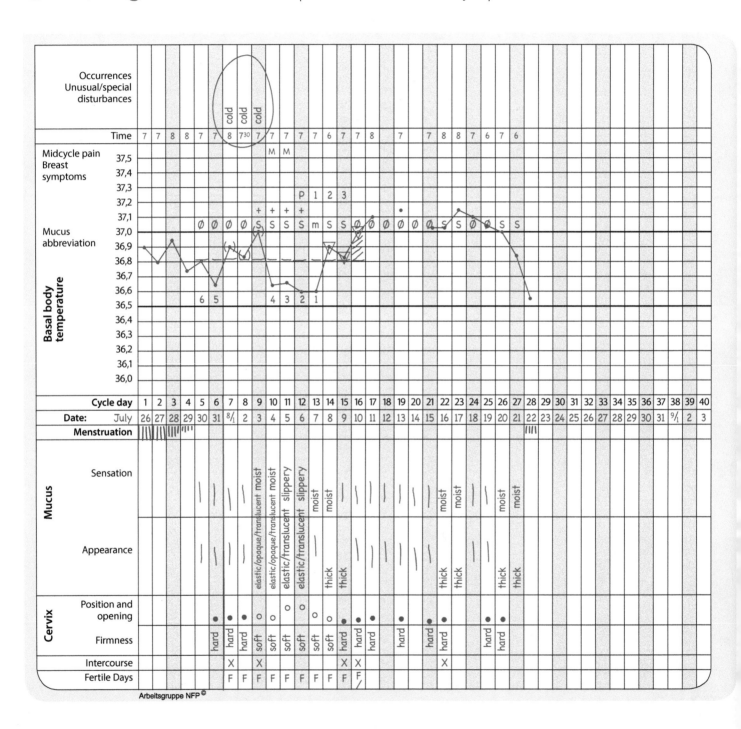

Arbeitsgruppe NFP ©

Cycle-no* | 1 | 7 |

®

Temperature taken
R X
V ☐
O ☐

Earliest first higher temperature reading in the previous cycles
| 1 | 4 |

Minus 8
| | 6 |

Earliest first higher temperature reading in this cycle
| 1 | 4 |

Do you intend to become pregnant in the next cycle?

yes X
no ☐
undecided ☐

✖ Malteser
...weil Nähe zählt.

Trying to conceive

1. The infertile time at the beginning of the cycle is identified using the Minus-8 Rule in double check with the cervical mucus sign. The last infertile day is cycle day 6. The infertile time after ovulation begins on the evening of cycle day 16.

2. On cycle days 7, 8, and 9, a cold affected temperature measurements and are considered disturbances. These values are put in brackets and not taken into account in the temperature shift evaluation.

3. Cristina L. has observed many signs of high fertility including mid-cycle pain, elastic and transparent cervical mucus, and a cervix that is soft, open, and high. However, she had intercourse only once at the beginning of the highly fertile time when she observed the highest quality cervical mucus.

Training 26b Special life circumstances and cycle patterns

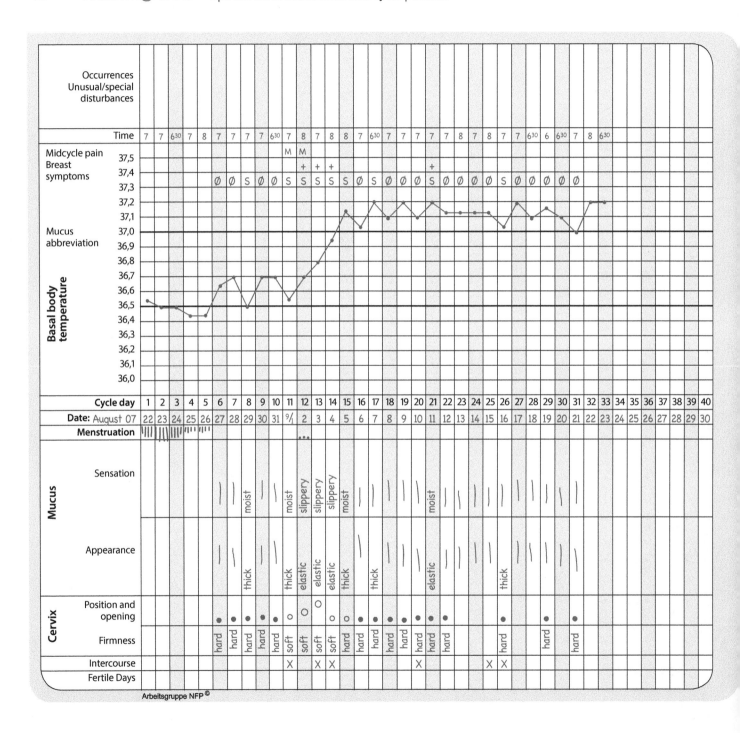

Occurrences Unusual/special disturbances

| Time | 7 | 7 | 6³⁰ | 7 | 8 | 7 | 7 | 7 | 7 | 6³⁰ | 7 | 8 | 7 | 8 | 8 | 7 | 6³⁰ | 7 | 7 | 7 | 7 | 8 | 7 | 8 | 7 | 7 | 6³⁰ | 6 | 6³⁰ | 7 | 8 | 6³⁰ | | | |

Midcycle pain / Breast symptoms — Mucus abbreviation — Basal body temperature

Temperature scale: 37,5 · 37,4 · 37,3 · 37,2 · 37,1 · 37,0 · 36,9 · 36,8 · 36,7 · 36,6 · 36,5 · 36,4 · 36,3 · 36,2 · 36,1 · 36,0

Midcycle pain markers: M M (days 12–13); Breast + (days 12, 13, 14, 21)

Mucus abbreviation row: Ø Ø S Ø Ø S S S S S S Ø S Ø Ø Ø S Ø Ø Ø Ø S Ø Ø Ø Ø Ø

Cycle day	1	2	3	4	5	6	7	8	9	10	11	12	13	14	15	16	17	18	19	20	21	22	23	24	25	26	27	28	29	30	31	32	33	34	35	36	37	38	39	40
Date: August 07	22	23	24	25	26	27	28	29	30	31	9/1	2	3	4	5	6	7	8	9	10	11	12	13	14	15	16	17	18	19	20	21	22	23	24	25	26	27	28	29	30

Menstruation: days 1–5 marked

Mucus

Sensation: (day 8) moist, (day 11) moist, (day 12) slippery, (day 13) slippery, (day 14) slippery, (day 15) moist, (day 21) moist

Appearance: (day 8) thick, (day 11) thick, (day 12) elastic, (day 13) elastic, (day 14) elastic, (day 15) thick, (day 17) thick, (day 21) elastic, (day 26) thick

Cervix

Position and opening: days 6–10 ● (closed); day 11 ○; day 12 ○ (raised); day 13 ○; day 14 ○; day 15 ○; days 16–21 ●; day 26 ●; day 29 ●; day 30 ●

Firmness: (6) hard (7) hard (8) hard (9) hard (10) hard (11) soft (12) soft (13) soft (14) soft (15) hard (16) hard (17) hard (18) hard (19) hard (20) hard (21) hard (26) hard (29) hard (30) hard

Intercourse: X on days 11, 13, 14, 20, 25, 26

Fertile Days:

Arbeitsgruppe NFP ©

SENSIPLAN ®

| Cycle-no* | | 1 | 8 |

Temperature taken

R X
V
O

Earliest first higher temperature reading in the previous cycles

Minus 8

Earliest first higher temperature reading in this cycle

Do you intend to become pregnant in the next cycle?

yes X
no
undecided

✠ **Malteser**
...weil Nähe zählt.

Trying to conceive

» **This is Cristina L.'s 18th cycle.**

1. Identify the beginning and end of the fertile time and mark this phase with "F."

2. Are there any disturbances or special circumstances?

3. What do you notice?

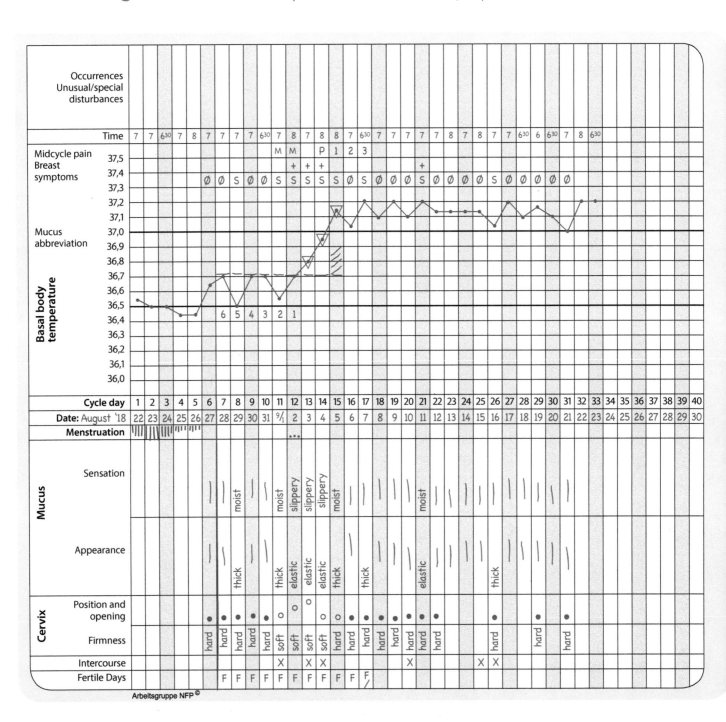

Arbeitsgruppe NFP ©

| Cycle-no* | 1 | 8 |

Temperature taken

R   X

V   ☐

O   ☐

Earliest first higher
temperature reading
in the previous cycles

| 1 | 4 |

Minus 8   6

Earliest first higher
temperature
reading in
this cycle

| 1 | 3 |

Do you intend to
become pregnant
in the next cycle?

yes   X

no   ☐

undecided   ☐

✳ Malteser
...weil Nähe zählt.

Trying to conceive

1. The infertile time at the beginning of the cycle is identified using the Minus-8 Rule in double check with the cervical mucus sign. The last infertile day is cycle day 6. The infertile time after ovulation begins on the evening of cycle day 17.

2. No disturbances or special circumstances are recorded.

3. Cristina L. has taken advantage of her highly fertile days (cycle days 11, 13, and 14) to have intercourse, and she conceived.

4. A temperature shift lasting more than 18 days and the absence of vaginal bleeding are indicators of pregnancy.

The probable due date is calculated as follows:

9/3/2018		8/27/2018		5/27/2018
– 7 Days		– 3 Months		+ 1 Year
= **8/27/2018**		= **5/27/2018**		= 5/27/2019

Basal body temperature scale (°C): 37,5 · 37,4 · 37,3 · 37,2 · 37,1 · 37,0 · 36,9 · 36,8 · 36,7 · 36,6 · 36,5 · 36,4 · 36,3 · 36,2 · 36,1 · 36,0

Occurrences / Unusual/special disturbances: "almost no sleep" (Cycle day 9)

Cycle day	1	2	3	4	5	6	7	8	9	10	11	12	13	14	15	16	17	18	19	20	21	22	23	24	25	26	27	28	29	30	31	32	33	34	35	36	37	38	39	40
Time	7	6	7	5	6³⁰	7	7	7	6³⁰	6	6	7	7	6	7³⁰	/	6	7	7	7	6¹⁵	6	7	7³⁰	6	6	7	7	6	6³⁰	7³⁰	6	6	7						
Date: October	13	14	15	16	17	18	19	20	21	22	23	24	25	26	27	28	29	30	31	11/1	2	3	4	5	6	7	8	9	10	11	12	13	14	15	16	17	18	19	20	21
Menstruation	∭	∭	∭	∭	∭	∭	∥																									∭								
Mucus – Sensation								moist	moist	moist	moist	moist	moist	moist	moist	moist	moist	moist	moist	moist	moist	moist	moist	moist	moist	moist	moist	moist	moist	moist	moist	moist								
Mucus – Appearance								whitish	whitish	whitish	elastic	elastic	elastic	whitish	stretchy	stretchy	stretchy	thick	thick	thick	thick	thick	thick	yellowish	yellowish	yellowish	yellowish	yellowish	yellowish	yellowish	thick	thick								
Cervix – Position and opening																																								
Cervix – Firmness																																								
Intercourse																																								
Fertile Days																																								

Row labels at left: Midcycle pain / Breast symptoms; Mucus abbreviation; Basal body temperature

Arbeitsgruppe NFP ©

SENSIPLAN ®

Cycle-no* [ ] 1

Postpartum

Temperature taken
R [X]
V [ ]
O [ ]

Weaning

Earliest first higher temperature reading in the previous cycles

[/]

Minus 8 [ ]

Earliest first higher temperature reading in this cycle [ ]

Do you intend to become pregnant in the next cycle?

yes [ ]
no [X]
undecided [ ]

✳ **Malteser**
...weil Nähe zählt.

Breastfeeding

» Lea B. is a 29-year-old mom; she recently stopped breastfeeding her seven-month-old baby. She is observing her first cycle since giving birth and stopping breastfeeding.

1. Identify the beginning and end of the fertile time and mark this phase with "F."

2. Are there any disturbances or special circumstances?

3. What do you notice?

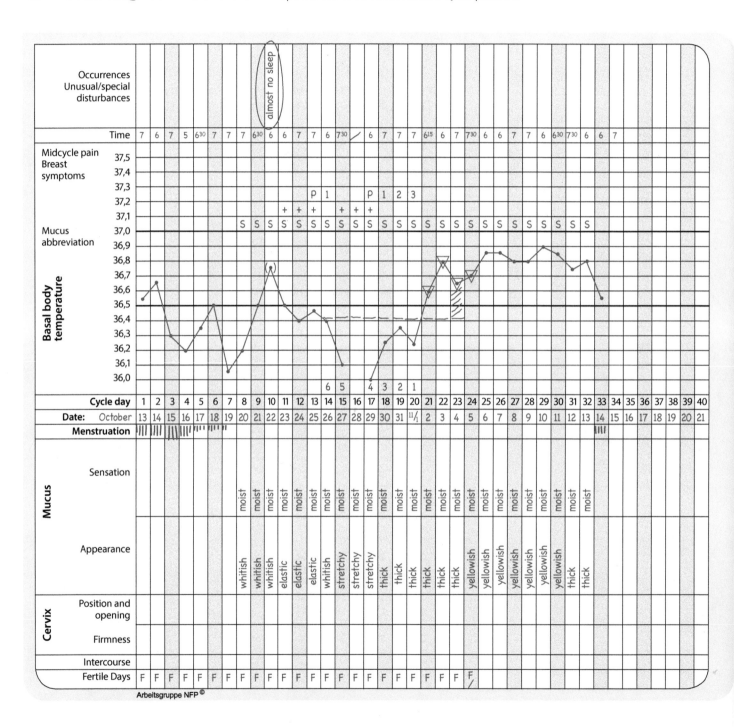

Arbeitsgruppe NFP ©

Breastfeeding

1. Since this is Lea B.'s first cycle using Sensiplan, the fertile time begins on cycle day 1. Fertility ends on the evening of cycle day 24.

2. On cycle day 10, "almost no sleep" affected the temperature measurement and is counted as a disturbance. This value is put in brackets and not taken into account.

3. More than seven months after having her baby, Lea B. observes her first ovulation. This late return of fertility is closely related to breastfeeding, which is known to delay the first ovulation. Her ovulation was preceded by a clear change in the cervical mucus sign.

Note:
- To identify a temperature shift evaluation in the first cycle after giving birth and during breastfeeding, an additional higher temperature measurement is required.

Cycle-no* | | 1 |

Postpartum

Temperature taken
R | X |
V | |
O | |

Weaning

Earliest first higher temperature reading in the previous cycles

Minus 8 | | |

Earliest first higher temperature reading in this cycle | 2 | 1 |

Do you intend to become pregnant in the next cycle?

yes | |
no | X |
undecided | |

Malteser
...weil Nähe zählt.

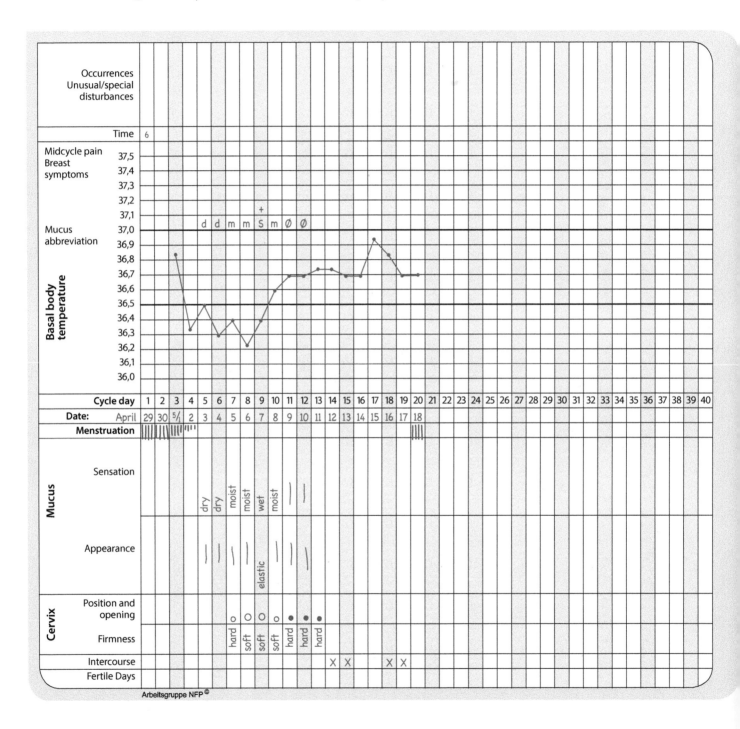

Arbeitsgruppe NFP ©

Cycle-no*   8   4

Temperature taken
   R ☐
   V ☐
   O ☒

Earliest first higher
temperature reading
in the previous cycles

      1   0

Minus 8   ☐☐

Earliest first higher
temperature
reading in
this cycle   ☐☐

Do you intend to
become pregnant
in the next cycle?

     yes ☐
     no ☐
  undecided ☐

Perimenopause

» **Regina M. is a 47-year-old teacher. She has two children and has been using Sensiplan for seven years.**

There was a temperature shift in the previous cycle.

1. Identify the beginning and end of the fertile time and mark this phase with "F."

2. Are there any disturbances or special circumstances?

3. What do you notice?

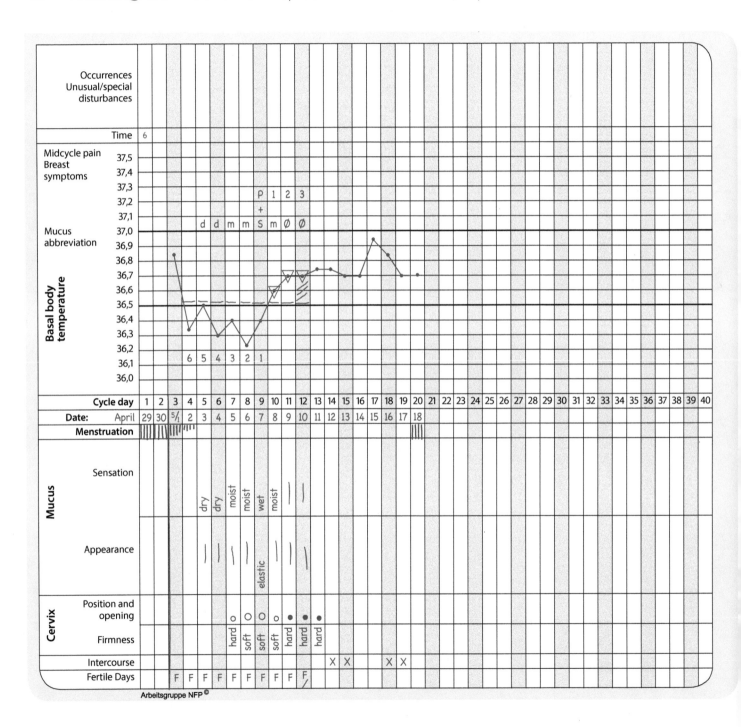

Arbeitsgruppe NFP ©

®

Cycle-no* | 8 | 4

Temperature taken

R ☐
V ☐
O ☒

Earliest first higher
temperature reading
in the previous cycles

| 1 | 0 |

Minus 8 | 2 |

Earliest first higher
temperature
reading in
this cycle

| 1 | 0 |

Do you intend to
become pregnant
in the next cycle?

yes ☐
no ☐
undecided ☐

Perimenopause

1. The infertile time at the beginning of the cycle is identified using the Minus-8 Rule in double check with the cervical mucus sign. The last infertile day at the beginning of the cycle is cycle day 2. The fertile time ends on the evening of cycle day 12.

2. No disturbances or special circumstances are recorded. However, Regina M. noticed the appearance of the cervical mucus sign on only four days.

3. Regina M.'s follicular phase was short, which caused a shortened cycle length. Cycles that get progressively shorter with early temperature shifts and a normal luteal phase length are typical during perimenopause.

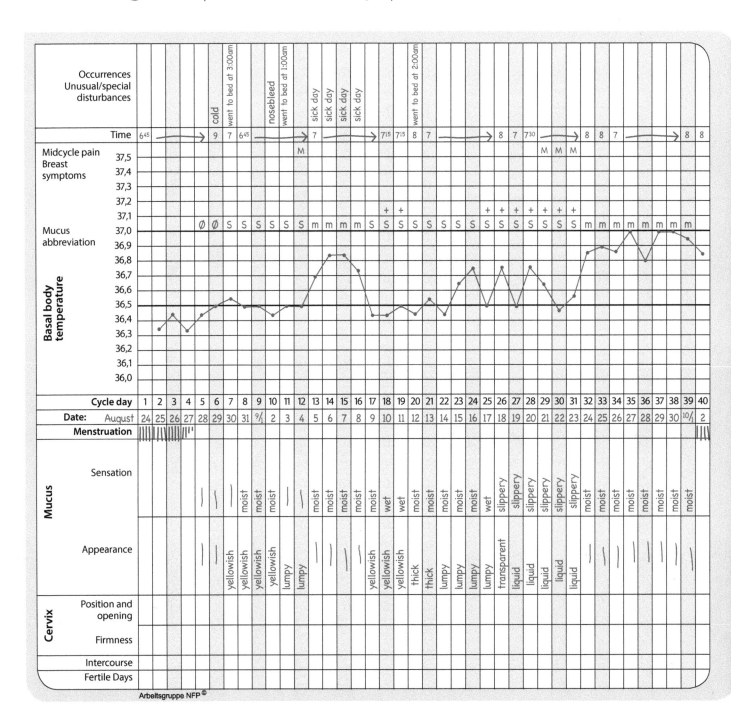

SENSIPLAN ®

Cycle-no* [ ] 1

Post pill

Temperature taken
R [ ]
V [X]
O [ ]

Earliest first higher
temperature reading
in the previous cycles

[/]

Minus 8 [ ]

Earliest first higher
temperature
reading in
this cycle [ ]

Do you intend to
become pregnant
in the next cycle?

yes [ ]
no [X]
undecided [ ]

✳ **Malteser**
...weil Nähe zählt.

After discontinuing hormonal contraceptives

» Lisa P. is a 28-year-old florist who has been on the pill for several years. She has decided to stop taking the pill and to learn Sensiplan.

Trainings 29a and 29b are the first two cycles after stopping the pill.

1. Identify the beginning and end of the fertile time and mark this phase with "F."

2. Are there any disturbances or special circumstances?

3. What do you notice?

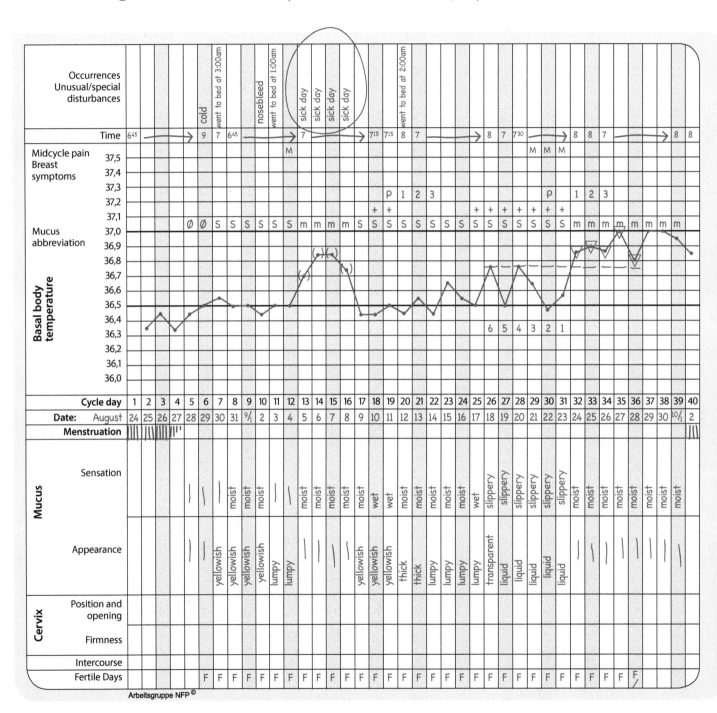

Arbeitsgruppe NFP ©

After discontinuing hormonal contraceptives

1. In the first cycle after discontinuing hormonal contraceptives, the first 5 cycle days are infertile. Because the temperature shift was evaluated using the first exception to the rule, and because this cycle was the first cycle since discontinuing hormonal contraception, two additional temperature measurements are required to complete the temperature shift evaluation.

2. On cycle days 13-16, "sick day" resulted in four days of temperature measurement increases and is counted as a disturbance. These values were put in brackets and not taken into account when evaluating the temperature shift. Other events, such as "cold," "nosebleed," or "went to bed late" had no effect on her temperature measurements and were not counted as disturbances. There are many days the cervical mucus sign is observed. There are two shifts in the cervical mucus sign.

3. The follicular phase is prolonged, while the luteal phase is short (8 days). This is a common observation in the first few cycles after discontinuing hormonal contraception. Sometimes no temperature shift at all is observed in the cycles immediately after discontinuing hormonal contraception (monophasic or anovulatory cycles). The long cervical mucus pattern with more than one shift is also common after discontinuing the pill.

®

Cycle-no* | | 1

Post pill

Temperature taken
R | |
V | X
O | |

Earliest first higher temperature reading in the previous cycles | /

Minus 8 | /

Earliest first higher temperature reading in this cycle | 3 | 2

Do you intend to become pregnant in the next cycle?

yes | |
no | X
undecided | |

Malteser
...weil Nähe zählt.

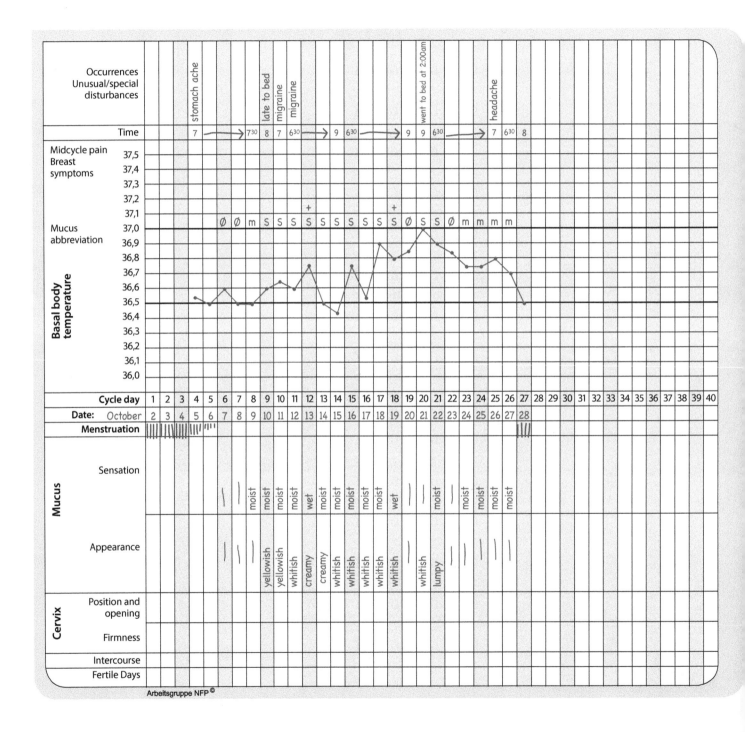

Occurrences Unusual/special disturbances		stomach ache; late to bed; migraine; migraine; went to bed at 2:00am; headache
Time		7 → 7³⁰ 8 7 6³⁰ → 9 6³⁰ → 9 9 6³⁰ → 7 6³⁰ 8

Midcycle pain
Breast symptoms

Mucus abbreviation: Ø Ø m S S S S S S S S S S S Ø S S Ø m m m m

(Breast symptom "+" marks at cycle day 12 and cycle day 18, row 37,1)

Basal body temperature

Temperature scale: 37,5 37,4 37,3 37,2 37,1 37,0 36,9 36,8 36,7 36,6 36,5 36,4 36,3 36,2 36,1 36,0

Cycle day	1	2	3	4	5	6	7	8	9	10	11	12	13	14	15	16	17	18	19	20	21	22	23	24	25	26	27	28	29	30	31	32	33	34	35	36	37	38	39	40
Date: October	2	3	4	5	6	7	8	9	10	11	12	13	14	15	16	17	18	19	20	21	22	23	24	25	26	27	28													
Menstruation	‖‖‖ ‖‖‖ ‖‖ ‖‖‖ ‖‖ ‖‖‖																					‖‖‖ ‖																			

Mucus

Sensation: moist moist moist moist wet moist moist moist moist moist wet moist moist moist moist moist

Appearance: yellowish yellowish whitish creamy creamy whitish whitish whitish whitish whitish whitish lumpy

Cervix

Position and opening

Firmness

Intercourse

Fertile Days

Arbeitsgruppe NFP ©

sensiplan ®	
Cycle-no*	2
Temperature taken	R
	V X
	O
Earliest first higher temperature reading in the previous cycles	
Minus 8	
Earliest first higher temperature reading in this cycle	
Do you intend to become pregnant in the next cycle?	
yes	
no	X
undecided	

✠ Malteser
...weil Nähe zählt.

After discontinuing hormonal contraceptives

» **This is Lisa P.'s next cycle.**

1. Identify the beginning and end of the fertile time and mark this phase with "F."

2. Are there any disturbances or special circumstances?

3. What do you notice?

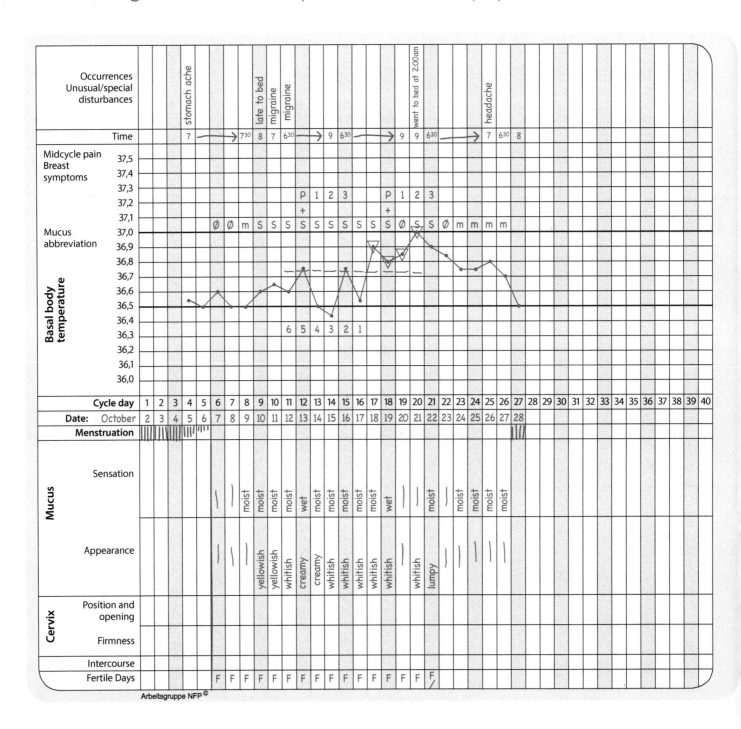

Arbeitsgruppe NFP ©

®

Cycle-no* 2

Temperature taken

R [ ]

V [X]

O [ ]

Earliest first higher temperature reading in the previous cycles 32

Minus 8 [/]

Earliest first higher temperature reading in this cycle 17

Do you intend to become pregnant in the next cycle?

yes [ ]

no [X]

undecided [ ]

Malteser
...weil Nähe zählt.

After discontinuing hormonal contraceptives

1. The infertile time at the beginning of the cycle was identified using the 5-Day Rule in double check with the cervical mucus sign. The last infertile day at the beginning of the cycle is cycle day 5. The infertile time after ovulation begins on the evening of cycle day 21.
2. Since "stomach ache," "late to bed," "migraines," and "headache" did not affect the temperature measurements, they are not counted as disturbances and are not put in brackets.
3. Similar to the previous cycle, there are two shifts in the cervical mucus sign. The second cervical mucus shift occurring on cycle day 18 is used to complete the evaluation because "S+" mucus was observed during the temperature shift.
4. The follicular phase length (16 days) and the luteal phase length (10 days) are beginning to return to normal lengths.

Note:

- The temperature shift is evaluated using the first exception to the rule.

Occurrences Unusual/special disturbances					late to bed	late to bed											late to bed	late to bed																							
Time	7				9	7											9	9																							

Midcycle pain / Breast symptoms / Mucus abbreviation

Basal body temperature

Cycle day	1	2	3	4	5	6	7	8	9	10	11	12	13	14	15	16	17	18	19	20	21	22	23	24	25	26	27	28	29	30	31	32	33	34	35	36	37	38	39	40
Date: May	3	4	5	6	7	8	9	10	11	12	13	14	15	16	17	18	19	20	21	22	23	24	25	26	27	28	29	30	31	6/1	2	3	4	5	6	7	8	9	10	11
Menstruation	||| ||| ||| ||| |||																							|||										

Mucus

| Sensation | | | | | | | moist | moist | moist | moist | moist | moist | slippery | moist | moist | wet | wet | wet | moist | moist | moist | | | | | | | | | | | | | | | | | | | |

| Appearance | | | | | | | thick | thick | thick | thick | elastic | translucent | thick | like egg white | | | whitish | thick | | | | | | | | | | | | | | | | | | | | | | |

Cervix

Position and opening				●	●					o	o			o	◯	◯◯	o	●																						
Firmness				hard	hard				soft	soft			soft	soft	soft	soft	hard																							
Intercourse			X	X															X		X																			
Fertile Days																																								

Arbeitsgruppe NFP ©

SENSIPLAN ®	
Cycle-no*		1	1	
Temperature taken	R X
	V
	O
Earliest first higher temperature reading in the previous cycles		1	2	
Minus 8		
Earliest first higher temperature reading in this cycle		
Do you intend to become pregnant in the next cycle?	
yes	
no	X
undecided	

✠ **Malteser**
...weil Nähe zählt.

And finally... Sensiplan in practice!

» **Lakshmi is a wardrobe director and is currently in her 11th cycle using Sensiplan. She does not have children.**

There was a temperature shift in the previous cycle.

1. Identify the beginning and end of the fertile time and mark this phase with "F."

2. Are there any disturbances or special circumstances?

3. What do you notice?

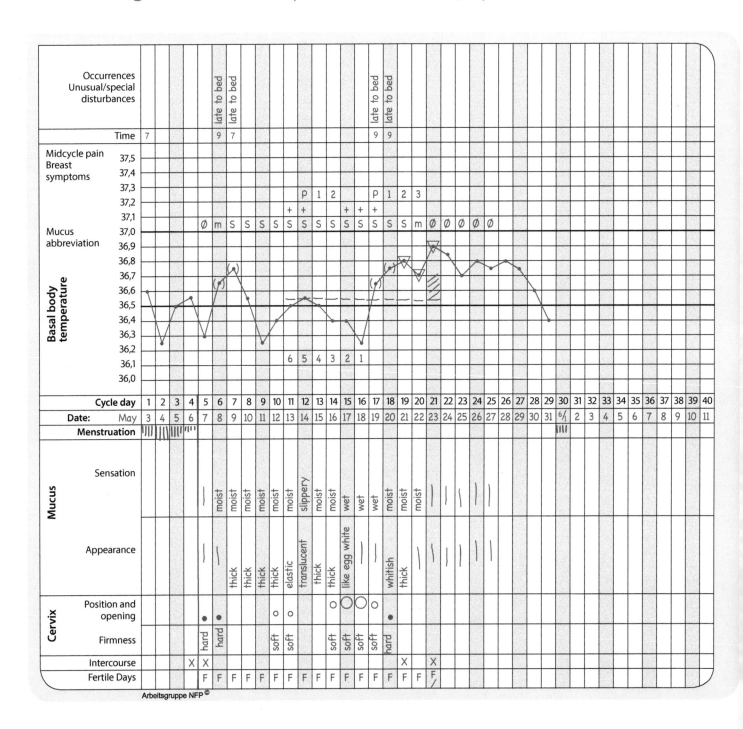

Arbeitsgruppe NFP ©

®

| Cycle-no* | 1 | 1 |

Temperature taken
R [X]
V [ ]
O [ ]

Earliest first higher
temperature reading
in the previous cycles

| 1 | 2 |

Minus 8 | 4 |

Earliest first higher
temperature
reading in
this cycle | 1 | 9 |

Do you intend to
become pregnant
in the next cycle?

yes [ ]
no [X]
undecided [ ]

❋ Malteser
...weil Nähe zählt.

And finally... Sensiplan in practice!

1. The infertile time at the beginning of the cycle is identified using the Minus-8 Rule in double check with the cervical mucus sign. The last infertile day is cycle day 4. The infertile time after ovulation begins on the evening of cycle day 21.

   Although Lakshmi has not completed 12 cycles of using Sensiplan, she uses the Minus-8 Rule instead of the 5-Day Rule because in a previous cycle she observed an earliest first higher temperature reading on cycle day 12.

2. On cycle days 6, 7, 17, and 18, "late to bed" affected the temperature measurement and are counted as disturbances. These values are put in brackets and not taken into account when evaluating the temperature shift.

3. There are two shifts in the cervical mucus sign. The second cervical mucus shift occurring on cycle day 17 is used to complete the evaluation.

4. Although she is not trying to conceive, Lakshmi had intercourse during the fertile time, on cycle days 5 and 19.

Infertile time at the beginning of the cycle

» If you would also like to identify the infertile time at the beginning of the cycle in Chapter 2, the solutions are provided here: *(All solutions assume a temperature shift in the previous cycle.)*

Training 8: The infertile phase at the beginning of the cycle was identified using the 5-Day Rule in double check with the cervical mucus sign. The last infertile day is cycle day 5.

Training 9: The infertile phase at the beginning of the cycle is identified using the Minus-8 Rule in double check with the cervical mucus sign. The last infertile day is cycle day 6.

Training 10: The infertile phase at the beginning of the cycle is identified using the Minus-8 Rule in double check with the cervical mucus sign. The last infertile day is cycle day 5.

Training 11: The infertile phase at the beginning of the cycle is identified using the Minus-8 Rule in double check with the cervical mucus sign. The last infertile day is cycle day 8.

Training 12: The infertile phase at the beginning of the cycle was identified using the 5-Day Rule in double check with the cervical mucus sign. The last infertile day is cycle day 5.

Training 13: The infertile phase at the beginning of the cycle was identified using the 5-Day Rule in double check with the cervical mucus sign. The last infertile day is cycle day 5.

Training 14: The infertile phase at the beginning of the cycle is identified using the Minus-8 Rule in double check with the cervical mucus sign. The last infertile day is cycle day 6.

Training 15: The infertile phase at the beginning of the cycle is identified using the Minus-8 Rule in double check with the cervical mucus sign. The last infertile day is cycle day 5.

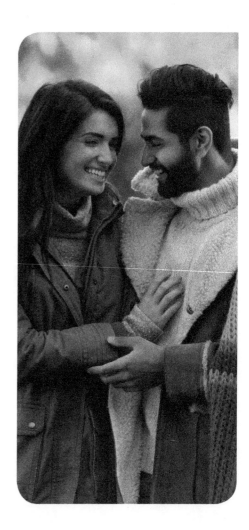

The Cervical Mucus Sign

» Making cervical mucus observations requires you to feel, see, and touch your cervical mucus throughout the day and evening. At the end of the day enter the best cervical mucus quality observed on the rows marked "Mucus."

Table 1: Cervical mucus classifications, observations and abbreviations

Feel/Touch		Appearance	Code
dry, rough, itching, unpleasant feeling	and	no visible mucus, no cervical mucus at the vaginal opening	▷ d
no mucus felt, no moistness, presence of mucus not sensed at the vaginal opening	and	no visible mucus, no cervical mucus at the vaginal opening	▷ ø
moist	but	no visible mucus, no cervical mucus at the vaginal opening	▷ m
moist but presence of mucus not sensed	and	thick, whitish, opaque, creamy, lumpy, yellowish, sticky, milky, non-elastic or tough	▷ S
moist, but presence of mucus not sensed	and	translucent, transparent, translucent sheen like raw egg white (translucent with white streaks), elastic or stretchy, can be stretched into strands, so liquid that it "runs like water", reddish, red-brown, yellowish-red	+ ▷ S
wet, slimy, slippery, lubricating, like oil, smooth	and/or	translucent, transparent, translucent sheen like raw egg white (translucent with white streaks), elastic or stretchy, can be stretched into strands, so liquid that it "runs like water", reddish, red-brown, yellowish-red	+ ▷ S

Evaluating cervical mucus observations

Rule: Shift of the cervical mucus sign - The cervical mucus shift is the last day of your best quality cervical mucus before it shifts to a lower quality. Determining the day of this shift (Peak day) can only be done after it has happened. On the chart below, the letter "P" shows the Peak day, or the last day of the best quality cervical mucus before the shift to a lower quality.

How is the cervical mucus sign evaluated?

First, determine the last day of your best quality cervical mucus before it shifts to a lower quality and mark it with a "P" above the cervical mucus abbreviation. Then mark the next three days as 1 - 2 - 3 (cf. *Natural & Safe: The Handbook*).

	Time																			
Midcycle pain Breast symptoms	37,5																			
	37,4																			
	37,3												P	1	2	3				
	37,2																			
	37,1									+	+	+								
Mucus abbreviation	37,0					d	m	s	s	s	s	s	s	s	ø	ø	d	d		
	36,9																			
	36,8																			
	36,7																			

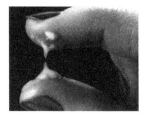

Whitish, creamy (S)

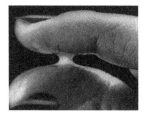

Milky or cloudy, tough elastic (S)

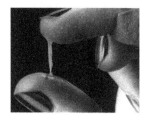

Whitish or yellowish, some tough elastic (S)

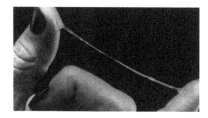

Translucent, stretchy (S+)

The Basal Body Temperature Sign

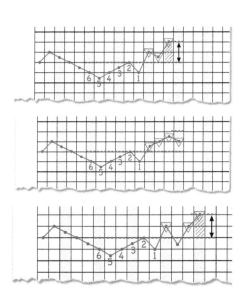

» How to measure your temperature

- Immediately after waking and before getting out of bed
- After at least one hour of rest or sleep
- Ideally every day
- By using an analog basal body thermometer or a calibrated digital thermometer displaying two decimal points
- Always use the same method: orally, rectally or vaginally (hold for 3 minutes); never under the arm

Table 2: Rounding off with a digital thermometer

Refer to the table on page 25 and the examples below to determine how to round (up or down) individual temperatures taken.

36.50 = 36.50	36.53 = 36.55	36.58 = 36.60
36.51 = 36.50	36.54 = 36.55	36.59 = 36.60
36.52 = 36.50	36.55 = 36.55	36.60 = 36.60
	36.56 = 36.55	
	36.57 = 36.55	

Evaluating temperature measurements

Rule: Temperature shift - A temperature shift can be confirmed when three consecutive readings are all higher than the six previous readings, and the 3rd higher reading is at least 2 boxes (2/10°C) above the previous six low-temperature readings.

First exception to the rule on temperature: If the 3rd temperature measurement is not 2/10 °C higher than the cover line, a 4th temperature measurement must be used. This also must be higher than the cover line, but it does not necessarily have to be 2/10°C higher.

Second exception to the rule on temperature: Out of three required higher temperature measurements, one measurement may fall down to or below the cover line. This value must not be taken into account and is therefore not triangled. The third value, however, must be at least 2/10 °C (2 boxes) above the cover line.

Note: The first and second exceptions to the rule cannot be used together in the same cycle.

The Optional Cervix Sign

» How is the cervix examined?

- Once a day
- In the same position and always with the same finger
- In a slightly stooped position

» What is assessed?

- The width of the opening of the cervix (closed, partially open, completely open)
- The position (lower/higher)
- The firmness (hard or soft)

Evaluating cervix observations

Rule: Cervix - If you choose to use the cervix sign instead of the cervical mucus sign, the infertile time after ovulation begins on the evening of the third day with a closed and hard cervix, using a double check with temperature measurements (cf. *Natural & Safe: The Handbook*)

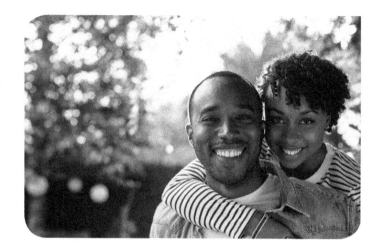

Cervix														
Appearance														
Position and opening				•	•	•	○	○	○	○	1	2	3
Firmness				hard	hard	hard	soft	soft	soft	soft	hard	hard	hard
Intercourse														
Fertile Days														

Double Check Rules

The 5-Day Rule

The first 5 cycle days can be assumed to be infertile days unless cervical mucus is noted or the Minus-8 Rule begins fertility first.

During your previous 12 cycles, if the earliest first higher temperature reading has ever been on or before cycle day 12, "the first 5 days of infertility" no longer applies. From that point on, the "earliest first higher temperature reading "Minus-8" Rule will apply.

The Minus-8 Rule

The last infertile day at the beginning of the cycle is the day of the earliest first higher temperature from at least 12 previous cycle charts minus-8 days.

If you observe cervical mucus or feel "moist," before this day, the fertile phase starts immediately using the double check principle of "whichever is first."

The Minus-20 Rule

To use the Minus-20 Rule, find your shortest cycle length from at least 12 previous cycles and subtract 20 days to identify your last infertile day at the beginning of the cycle.

If you observe cervical mucus before this day, the fertile phase starts immediately using the double check principle of "whichever is first."

CPSIA information can be obtained
at www.ICGtesting.com
Printed in the USA
JSHW041628030520
5360JS00009B/10